How to Look and Feel Younger for Longer

With simple guidelines that work no matter what age or gender you are!

ELLEN JOUBERT

I dedicate this book to all the women and men whose desire is to improve their health and appearance, and to age gracefully. Lots of love, Ellen

ACKNOWLEDGEMENTS

Firstly, I want to thank God, who enabled me to have the time to write this second book. Secondly, I want to thank my family, who have supported me all the way on the journey while I was writing this book: my husband, Marius; my dad, Johan; my daughters, Ellen Jnr. and Maria. Thank you for the encouragement. I love you all!

Thanks also to my daughter Ellen Jnr., who has assisted me with her creative skills as a graphic designer by drawing and creating new images, giving me professional advice, and helping to take some of the photos for this book.

God bless you all!

Wife, daughter, and mother, Ellen Joubert

CONTENTS

FOREWORD

Our face conveys our image to the world. It tells the story of what is going on in our lives. Stress, bad habits, unhealthy eating, sickness, lack of confidence, and mistreatment of the skin are all attributes that people will observe when they look at our face. The face, eyes, neck, décolletage region and hair form our face that the world sees. William Shakespeare said 'The eyes are the window to the soul'. So your face reveals your whole life to the outside world. With the use of cosmetics, dress style and a beautiful hairstyle, we can successfully hide things from others. But it takes a bit more effort to make sure we maintain a healthy and attractive appearance throughout our lifetime, and not just through our youthful years.

Using good quality skin care products is essential to look younger for longer in your life, but skin care practices play an even bigger role in maintaining healthy and good-looking skin. This book is full of tips and techniques on how you can preserve youthful skin. The sooner a child starts to look after their skin, the longer they will have a beautiful skin, but it starts with their parents. I believe that every mother and father has an obligation to teach their kids from an early age to look after their face and overall skin condition.

One important fact that I would like to point out is that you do not need to be born with the most attractive features to look good and make a good impression. A well-cared-for face is what is essential to looking beautiful and attractive, and this can be achieved by anyone. It is not difficult to make yourself look attractive. All it takes is the knowledge about how to do it, and dedication. I acknowledge that we did not all learn how to effectively look after our faces and our skin.

Just as we cannot be all engineers or doctors, we cannot be all beauty therapists. We are there to help and support each other in what we have been trained in, and together we support each other, making life easier for one another. After I finished secondary school, I enrolled into a three year course of full-time study, and completed a beauty technology qualification in South Africa. I also completed an international qualification for beauty therapists called Comité International d'Esthétique et de Cosmétology, or C.I.D.E.S.C.O. Maybe you had the opportunity to study to be a beauty therapist like I did. But for the majority of people, they never had the chance to learn the proper ins and outs of skin care. You are lucky if your mother or grandmother had an impact in your life, teaching you about proper skin care. A lot of people make this out to be difficult, expensive or time consuming, when in fact, it should be a lifestyle. Just as you have to eat daily to stay alive and healthy, your face and skin require the right treatment to look, and stay healthy as well.

It's an awesome compliment to get when someone says to you that you have a beautiful skin. For those who do not have beautiful skin, this is ninety nine per cent correctable through the right treatment, diet and lifestyle practices. There are no excuses anymore to not feel beautiful or handsome. It is all about having the right knowledge and applying it. That is where I come in. I want to show you how easy it is to look admirable throughout your lifetime.

The right skin care program should really start from the time you are born. That is why I say good skin care practices starts with the mothers and fathers. Of course you'll not use the same skin care products on a baby and young children's skin, as you would on an adult's skin. Natural and simple formulas come into play, with the correct practices.

In addition, there is nothing feminine about skin care; men need to look after their face and skin as well to preserve it for longer. I have a lot of respect for a man who looks after his face and skin.

Ellen Joubert, your partner in looking
and feeling younger for longer.

THE IMPORTANCE OF LOOKING AFTER YOUR SKIN

It is extremely important to cleanse your face every day, morning and night. Splashing your face with water in the shower or in the washbasin isn't washing. You need a face cleanser that is not your normal bar of soap that you wash your hands with to cleanse your face and neck properly. This gives them a chance to rejuvenate and hydrate, and prevents possible bacterial invasion. Cleansing and caring for the skin correctly is not just to help you look younger for longer in life, it also keeps your overall skin healthy and free from any illnesses.

Research shows cleansing your face before going to bed at night is essential to looking younger for longer. I agree with the researchers because after qualifying as a beauty therapist in my early twenties, I used everything that I am teaching you in the skin care section now for many years, and I am reaping the benefits of it in my late forties. I can say with confidence that I practice what I preach.

Some people care more for the rest of their body by showering and getting rid of excreted skin oils and environmental debris every day, than looking after their face. As I have mentioned in the foreword, your 'face' includes your face, eyes, neck, décolletage region and hair. It can be seen that if only one of the above is not looked after, it can affect the total appearance of the face.

Ladies, those of you who wear a thick layer of make-up every day may have to cleanse your face twice at night to get rid of all the foundation and creams, to give the skin a proper chance to rejuvenate. Everything on this earth requires breathing to stay alive, and if you do not give your skin a chance to breathe at night, it will look dull. Another word for dull is lifeless.

While you are young and beautiful you may think: 'I do not need to put so much effort in because I am beautiful.' That is where you make the biggest mistake in your life, as no one stays young forever. We mature a bit more every day, and after the age of twenty-five years you'll one day notice that you have aged quite a bit. The reason is that from that point in your life your skin is starting to lose its youthful look and elasticity. In other words, the skin is slowly losing its ability to snap back after stretching. Think of an elastic band, when it is new you can keep stretching it and it will return to its original size every time. The more you stretch it, the more it gets stretched out, and will come to a point where it will stretch no more. It can even break when all the elasticity is worn out. All the damage and mistreatment to the skin in your earlier years will start to show from the age of twenty-five. For those who have mistreated their skin a lot, will see signs of wrinkles and the loss of elasticity sooner than their twenty-five years. Further on you'll learn how to treat the skin well in order for it to look younger for longer.

Although damaged skin cannot be repaired, it can be improved quite a bit with good practices and the right techniques. So it is never too late to start looking after your skin and face.

Our skin is aging and the simple process of cleansing our face before bed at night is an excellent way to mitigate the external factors associated with aging and to stimulate the internal processes that fight aging. We are washing the following off from our skin every night: sebum (that is a light yellow, oily substance secreted by the sebaceous glands in the skin to keep it naturally moisturised), environmental debris, sweat, creams and make-up. A tradesperson may even have elements of oil or dirt on their skin.

The most important reasons why you have to wash off all of the above substances from your skin every night are: to stop the working process of any bacteria and to give the skin a chance to rejuvenate, or renew. Human skin repairs itself during nighttime and requires oxygen for the repairing process. When we go to sleep with the skin's natural oil, creams, and make-up, we deprive the skin of this vital nutrient. Make-up, oils and creams also block the natural exfoliating process and will leave the skin looking dull. Forgoing regular nighttime cleansing will furthermore give you larger pores. When make-up and dirt is left on at night, it seeps deep down your skin, clogging pores.

Every night when you sleep on your pillow with an uncleansed face, the make-up and dirt rubs off on the pillow case. Imagine all the bacterial activity that occurs on your pillow that you expose your face to every night.

Washing your bed linen weekly is also crucial to get rid of all the sweat and dead skin that attracts dust mites and microscopic bugs that live on the fibres of your sheets. While dust mites eat your dead skin flakes, they are also excreting in your sheets; and their excrement has been known to cause asthma and allergies.

Sebaceous
gland

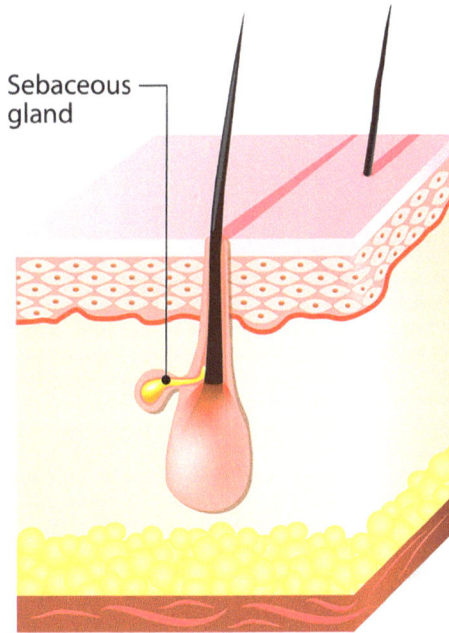

Illustration of the sebaceous gland producing sebum

Another component in the human skin that helps with elasticity and strength is collagen. Collagen is the most abundant protein in our bodies and is found in muscles, bones, skin, blood vessels, the digestive system and tendons. Along with the elasticity and strength it provides to your skin it also assists with the replacing of dead skin cells.

Researchers found that once your collagen levels start to decline due to the aging process, the face's skin pores do not snap back as easily once they become enlarged. Leaving make-up on when you go to bed at night then, can also lead to inflammation, which generates free radicals and collagen breakdown.

Just as your whole body requires daily cleansing to stop bacteria development and odours, your face requires the same treatment. The difference is that your face is every day exposed to nature's elements such as sun, wind and environmental debris. While your body gets some protection from the clothes you wear, your face is open and exposed to all the elements.

The skin of the face is more delicate compared to the rest of your body, and therefore requires special attention. You'll enhance the appearance of your skin and it will feel and look good for much longer in life by using the correct techniques and skin care products for your skin type. Even though men generally have a thicker skin than women, they need to look after their skin to maintain a healthier and younger looking skin during their lifetime.

Our face conveys our image to the world and if our face looks good it boosts our confidence and mental state. I promise you that you will feel and see a difference when you start looking after your face and skin the correct way. It saddens me when I see how some people neglect to look after their precious skin. The other misconception that some people have is that you need to use very expensive products to be able to keep your youthful look for longer. This cannot be further from the truth. We do not have to use the most expensive skin products on the market. Yes, there are some great products that can definitely make your skin appear so much younger, but we cannot all afford and maintain an expensive skin routine.

Consequently, the secret of looking younger for longer is to start early in life with a good face cleansing routine and hygienic habits, then maintain these through life. When we get to our forties and fifties, all the years of maintaining good face cleansing practices and habits will pay off big time. Not to mention all the years in between where you will look and feel good about yourself.

The same way people have different personalities, skins have different personalities too. Some people may have a sensitive skin, while others may have dry, oily, normal or problem skin. Different skin care products and different cleansing techniques are used to treat each individual skin type. A normal face cleansing routine should only take you two-three minutes in the morning and night to maintain a healthy-looking skin.

Our skin recovers overnight and therefore we will have more dead skin cells and sebum in the morning to wash off. This will require a face cleanser to wash it off successfully. Water alone removes only around sixty five per cent of oil and debris from the surface of the skin. Therefore you'll be leaving some debris and dirt behind if you only cleanse your face with water every day. So even though you have cleansed your face the night before, you'll have to cleanse it in the morning again to rid of the dead skin cells and sebum from the surface.

THE MEANING OF PH BALANCED

Normal hand and body soap is not suitable to use on the face, because it is too harsh for the delicate skin of the face. If you prefer soap rather than a milk or cream cleanser for your face, it is important to choose a soap that is pH Balanced and formulated specifically for the face. A soap bar or liquid soap that is pH balanced is not recommended for a dry skin though, as the skin will become drier over time. I'll reveal more through this book on which face cleanser is best for each skin type. You'll also discover your skin type further on.

It's not financially feasible to use the same skin care products that we use on our face, on the rest of the body. But we still have to make use of good skin care practices and techniques to retain good skin over the rest of our body too. Applying skin lotion over the rest of the body after each shower will preserve beautiful skin as well.

WE ONLY GET ONE SKIN IN LIFE, THEREFORE WE NEED TO DO
EVERYTHING WE CAN TO PROTECT AND PAMPER IT IN ORDER FOR
IT TO STAY HEALTHY AND YOUTHFUL FOR AS LONG AS POSSIBLE
THROUGHOUT OUR LIFETIME.

---

pH stands for 'potential of Hydrogen' and is a scale that measures acidity and alkalinity. Zero is the most acidic and fourteen the most alkaline, while seven is neutral, where water falls. The skin's natural pH hovers around five, and so is slightly acidic. This acidic environment supports growth of the skin's natural bacteria and fungus, which is necessary for proper skin health.

Our skin has a thin, protective layer on its surface, referred to as the acid mantle. This acid mantle is made up of sebum (free fatty acids) excreted from the skin's sebaceous glands, that mixes with lactic and amino acids from sweat to create the skin's pH, and ideally should be slightly acidic at about 5.5 on the pH scale.

Many factors can interfere with the delicate balance of the skin's acid mantle, both externally and internally. As we age, our skin becomes more acidic in response to our lifestyle and our environment. Everything that comes in contact with our skin such as products, smoking, air, water, sun and pollution, can contribute to the breaking down of the acid mantle, disrupting the skin's ability to protect itself.

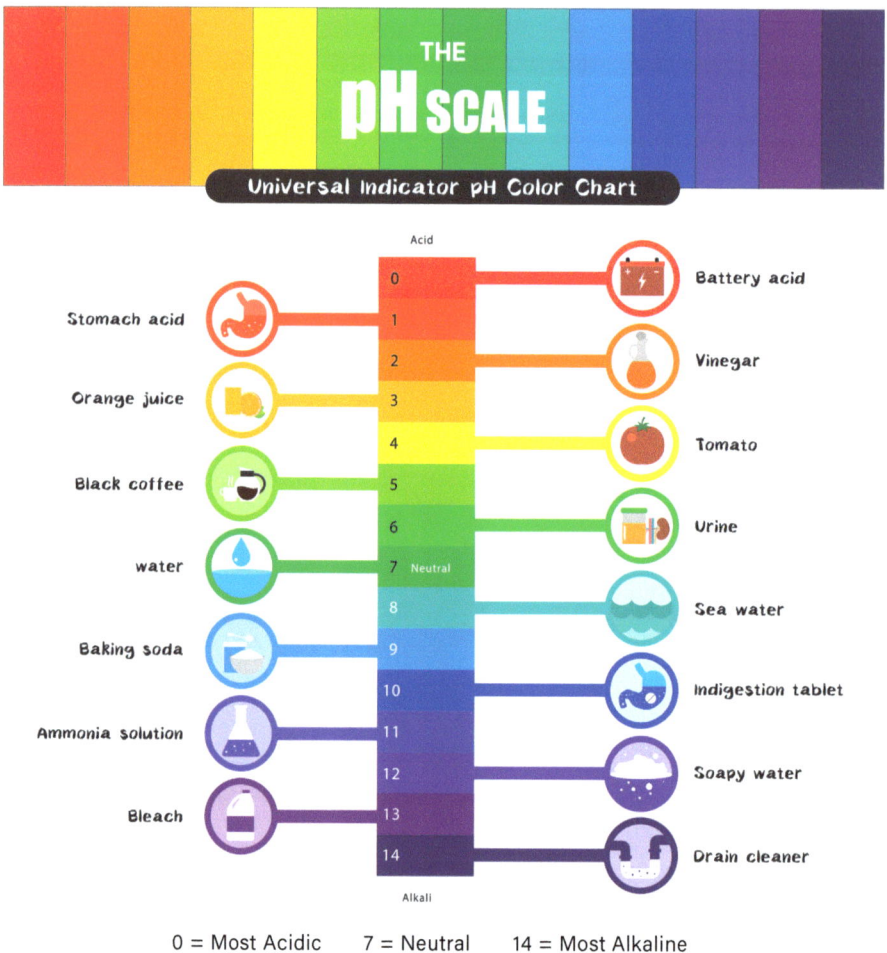

THE pH SCALE

Universal Indicator pH Color Chart

Acid

	pH	
Stomach acid	0	Battery acid
	1	
	2	Vinegar
Orange juice	3	
	4	Tomato
Black coffee	5	
	6	Urine
water	7 Neutral	
	8	Sea water
Baking soda	9	
	10	Indigestion tablet
Ammonia solution	11	
	12	Soapy water
Bleach	13	
	14	Drain cleaner

Alkali

0 = Most Acidic   7 = Neutral   14 = Most Alkaline

Maintaining the acid mantle of the skin

The acid mantle is an effective form of protection, but if the pH level is too alkaline or too acidic, the mantle is disturbed and skin conditions such as dermatitis, eczema and rosacea may result. A skin product may claim to be pH balanced, and then is not. You can verify the actual pH of a product by using an at-home pH testing kit, available at most pharmacies. A physician can determine your skin's surface pH level and a saliva test can accurately indicate your body's overall pH level.

Most face and neck cleansers, including soap bars and detergent soaps, tend to be too alkaline, and strip away the natural oils on the skin, causing dryness and irritation. A skin that is too alkaline can be more susceptible to acne because a certain level of acidity is needed to inhibit bacterial growth on the skin. Choosing mild cleansers and toners that are slightly acidic and close to five will benefit all skin types to properly maintaining the acid mantle.

Changing the pH of your skin

Before trying to change the pH of your skin look at your skin. Experiencing regular breakouts on an oily skin type means the pH of your skin is too acidic. Chronic dry skin or premature aging can mean your skin is too alkaline. Eliminate harsh cleansers like soaps that are alkaline, choose products that are rich in vitamins and antioxidants. Avoid products with hidden chemicals that harm the skin. Use only pH balanced products with a pH of 5.5. Cleanse and rinse the skin with lukewarm water instead of too warm water.

Distinctive features and functions of the skin

The human skin is the largest organ in the body and weighs around 3-4.5 kg (8-10 pounds) in an average adult. It's considered an organ because it meets the definition of a group of related cells that combine to perform one or more specific functions within the body, which is vital for survival and health of the body.

THE THREE LAYERS OF THE HUMAN SKIN

1. ***Epidermis****:* The outermost layer of skin that provides a waterproof barrier and creates our skin tone. This is the layer that we shed continuously.

2. ***Dermis:*** Is beneath the epidermis and contains tough connective tissue, hair follicles, and sweat glands. The dermis nourishes the epidermis.

3. ***Hypodermis:*** This layer is the deeper subcutaneous tissue below the dermis and is made up of fat cells and connective tissue supplied by blood vessels and the lymphatic system. The hypodermis supplies nutrients to the other two layers. It also cushions and insulates the body.

FEATURES OF THE SKIN

Our apparent lack of body hair immediately distinguishes human beings from all other large land mammals. Regardless of individual or racial differences, the human body seems to be more or less hairless, on the

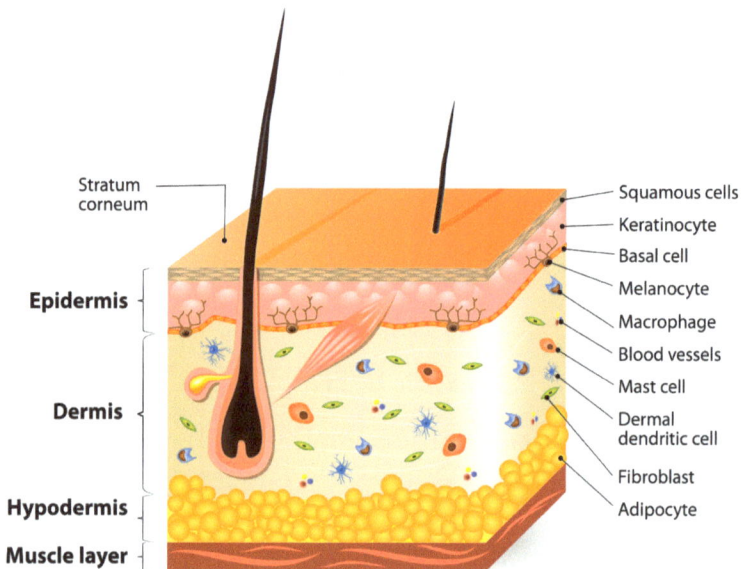

Illustration of the Human Skin

sense that the hair is as vestigial as to almost absent; yet in certain areas hair grows profusely. The characteristic features of skin change from the time of birth to old age. In infants and children it is velvety, dry, soft, and largely free of wrinkles and blemishes. Children younger than two years sweat poorly and irregularly; their sebaceous function is minimal. At adolescence hair becomes longer, thicker, and more pigmented, particularly in the scalp, armpits, pubic eminence, and the male face. General skin pigmentation increases, visible pigmentation spots appear mysteriously, and acne lesions often develop. Hair growth, sweating, and sebaceous secretions begin to blossom. As a person ages, anatomical and physiological alterations, as well as exposure to sunlight and wind, leave skin, particularly skin not protected by clothing, dry, wrinkled, and flaccid.

Human skin, more than that of any other mammal, exhibits striking topographic differences. An example is the dissimilarity between the palms and the backs of the hands and fingers. The skin of the eyebrows is thick, coarse, and hairy; and on the eyelids it is thin, smooth, and covered with almost invisible hairs. The face is seldom visibly haired on the forehead and cheekbones. It is completely hairless in the vermilion border of the lips, yet coarsely hairy over the chin and jaws of males.

The surfaces of the forehead, cheeks, and nose are normally oily, in contrast with the relatively greaseless lower surface of the chin and jaws. The skin of the chest, pubic region, scalp, armpits, abdomen, soles of the feet, and ends of the fingers varies as much structurally and functionally.

Differences do exist in structure and physiology of skin among different ethnicities and may differently influence disease. However, data on ethnic differences in skin physiology and function are few. The purpose of this book is for you to realise how important it is to look after your skin and not to give you a whole biology lesson. For this reason I'll not go in too much technical detail on the difference between the different skin colours, but just give enough information to help you understand the difference to choose the correct skin care products.

Firstly the major difference is the different skin colouring that ranges from the darkest brown to the lightest hues. An individual's skin pigmentation is the result of genetics, being the product of both of the individual's biological parents' genetic makeup. The single most important substance is the pigment melanin in the skin that is produced within the skin cells called melanocytes, and it's the major determinant of the skin colour of tanned to darker-skinned humans. The skin colour of people with light skin is determined mainly by the bluish-white connective tissue under the dermis and by the hemoglobin circulating in the veins of the dermis. The red colour underlying the skin becomes more visible, especially in the face, when, as consequence of physical exercise or the stimulation of the nervous system caused by anger and fear, when arterioles dilate. Colour is not entirely uniform across an individual's skin; for example, the skin of the palms and the soles is lighter than most other skin, and this is especially noticeable in tanned to darker-skinned people.

As the result of more melanin being present in tanned and darker skins, they have more protection against sun rays, as melanin protects the skin. Individuals with darker skin can be in the sun for longer than those with very light to lighter skin colours before they will sunburn. There is also a direct correlation between the geographic distribution of ultraviolet radiation (UVR) and the distribution of indigenous skin pigmentation around the world. Areas that receive higher amounts of UVR, generally located closer to the equator, tend to have darker-skinned populations. However, even though coloured skins by nature absorb up to thirty six per cent more solar radiation than the Caucasian skin, there is a lower incidence of sun-induced skin cancer in coloured skins. It can be concluded that melanin is a very efficient natural sunscreen.

Although melanin appears to be protective against the skin cancer forming properties of sunlight in darker skins, it does not protect against damage to the immune system. Regardless of skin colour, ultra violet rays (UVR) can suppress the skin's immune system by damaging the Langerhans cells and other skin barrier defence systems including Vitamin A deficiency, which will lead to skin ageing, pigmentation and enhance susceptibility to infection. Therefore darker skins will need to take the same precautions against UVR as individuals with lightly pigmented skin.

Researchers also found that darker skins are more sensitive to irritants and display a stronger skin irritant reaction than lighter skin, especially to the ingredient sodium lauryl sulfate that causes a significant increase in cutaneous blood flow in all skin colours and types. So check your skin products to make sure they do not include this ingredient.

Other differences between dark skin and light skin

- Dark skin has a higher electrical resistance than light skin, which suggests greater cohesion and thickness.

- Dark skin has more and larger fibroblasts (a cell in connective tissue which produces collagen and other fibres), than light skin. The fibroblasts in dark skin are also more multi-nucleated. This can lead to more abnormal scarring and keloid formation.

- The outermost layer of the skin (epidermis) of dark skins has more layers and stronger cells.

- Dark skin and Asian skin have a thicker and more compact dermis; this is why they are fortunate enough to have fewer facial wrinkles than the lighter skin.

- Dark skin has more casual lipids and more moisture in the epidermis.

- The pH level of the dark skin is also lower than light skins. Therefore the same products and treatment that are suitable for the light skin will not be suitable for darker skin.

After reading these obvious differences, read skin care product labels and instructions carefully to make sure you do not use skin products that will not contribute to the health of your skin. The major difference then between light, tanned and dark skins is duration of tolerance to sun exposure. Ideally you should use a skin care product formulated specifically for your skin colour and type, and of course the dark skin will appear younger for longer, if looked after. The rest of the information that follows regarding the functions of the skin, factors of skin aging, cleansing your skin the correct way, the different skin types, do's and don'ts in skin care, and correct cleansing steps, are exactly the same for all skin colours.

Just as we have differences in our colour of our teeth, eyes, and hair, we have differences in skin colours. As ethnic issues are still an unfortunate part of life, I want to encourage you to believe that we are all created uniquely and have to be proud of who we are. Look after your skin and appearance in a positive way. Let's age gracefully together just as we respect all uniquely created individuals together. No one can change who they were born to be, but we can change our appearance to look well cared for. I believe this is what makes the biggest difference in the world.

FUNCTIONS OF THE SKIN

- The skin protects most of the body's other vital organs, as well as its bones, muscles, ligaments and nerves, by acting as an envelope to contain them. Skin therefore forms a barrier and protects the organs from biological, chemical and mechanical attacks by outside forces, and combats infections. When the body experiences blood loss from a small cut or wound, the skin's healing properties help to constrain the blood loss by sealing the wound against infection and restoring tissue strength. The skin also protects the body from harmful sunrays and further damage.

- It helps to regulate the body's temperature through dissipating heat and sweating to bring the body's temperature back to a normal range, thus protecting the body against cold and against excessive amounts of water loss.

- It aids excretion of toxic substances through sweating. Dead skin cells on the surface of the epidermis layer are also a form of bodily waste that facilitates the growth of new epidermal cells. You lose around thirty thousand plus dead skin cells every minute that get replaced immediately by new skin tissue. The body does an excellent job of shedding dead skin cells through normal activity, but regular bathing or showering will serve as an accelerator.

- The sense of touch is dependent on the skin. The many nerve endings spreading throughout skin cells act to exchange information with the outside world, responding to touch, heat, cold and pain.

- It produces Vitamin D that is in fact a hormone. During exposure to sunlight, ultraviolet radiation penetrates the epidermis. The sun's energy turns a chemical in your skin into Vitamin D3 that is carried to your liver and then your kidneys transform it to active vitamin D. It keeps your bones healthy by increasing the intestinal absorption of calcium.

- The skin acts as a water-resistant barrier, so essential nutrients are not washed out of the body, and fluids do not enter the body through the skin.

- It gives us our unique skin colour.

- It allows stretching in the times of growth and continuous movement.

- The skin also forms the acid mantle that is a very fine, slightly acidic film on the surface of the skin acting as a barrier to bacteria, viruses and other potential contaminants that might penetrate the skin.

FACTORS OF SKIN AGING

Skin aging is divided into two categories, intrinsic and extrinsic.

Intrinsic factors

Skin aging factors that are not under your control.

Heredity: If one or both parents had good skin well into their old age, chances are you could inherit the same characteristics.

Hormones: The most dramatic changes in a woman's appearance take place around her menopause years when estrogen drops, causes considerable loss of collagen, which is an important protein that makes up most of the skin's supportive structure. As a result, wrinkles appear and skin hangs loosely.

Cellular recession: The process of aging originates on microscopic level. When numerous functions on cellular level are impaired, the cell cannot perform the metabolic and regenerating activities that promote health of the skin. These results in visible signs of aging are wrinkles, skin sagging and furrows.

Extrinsic factors

These are factors that you have control over. Fortunately the factors that have the biggest impact on skin aging are extrinsic which you can control to enhance the look of your skin and keep it younger for longer.

Sun exposure: Sunlight is the major factor of premature skin aging. According to the estimation of researchers, damage caused by ultraviolet rays of the sun is responsible for up to eighty per cent. The main reason why sunlight is so harmful to the skin is that it triggers free radical production in the skin that attacks the collagen. Most of the sun damage happens in the early part of our lives when our cheeks are still glowing with freshness of youth, but dramatic results do not appear until we are in our late thirties or forties.

Wear and tear: These are expression lines that appear on your face when you smile or frown. Over time this leaves a permanent stamp on your face. It is hard to avoid, but there is still something you can do about it, for example facial exercises and wrinkle relaxers.

Smoking: Decreases the flow of oxygen to the skin by as much as thirty per cent. Fine blood vessels in the dermis of the skin constrict, cutting off the supply of nutrients that are necessary for constant self-regeneration of the skin, and removal of waste products. As a result the skin begins to look grey and dull. Smoking also triggers the production of free radicals in the body. Besides of upsetting the balance of bodily tissue and organs, the free radicals attack collagen in the skin making it loses its elasticity and resilience.

Air pollution: Similarly to cigarette smoke, air pollutants restrict the flow of oxygen and nutrients to the skin and trigger excess free radical production. Free radicals are a by-product of normal metabolic activity and are always present in the body. When they are present within healthy norms, they are neutralised by built-in mechanisms of the body before wreaking havoc in your bodily tissues. The real problem begins when external factors like sunlight, cigarette smoke and pollution cause them to increase to the levels that your body is incapable of neutralising.

Lifestyle habits: These include eating habits, how much sleep you get every day, the degree of stress you are exposed to, the amount and type of exercise you engage in. Healthy habits slow progression of aging of your whole body, as well as your skin. Drinking six to eight glasses of water per day, cleansing and moisturising your skin daily, will slow down the aging process significantly.

Skin care products: Not using pH balanced products will make your skin too alkaline or too acidic. If your skin is too alkaline, it may be more prone to showing signs of premature ageing such as deep wrinkles, crow's feet and ultra violet damage. When a skin is too acidic, it can become inflamed, red and sore. To bring your skin back to the perfect balance, all you need to do is make sure that the products you apply to your skin are pH balanced. This means that the pH levels of your skin care products should sit around 4.5-6.

CLEANSING YOUR FACE THE CORRECT WAY

Washing your face seems pretty simple and easy as you have been doing it your whole life. But have you ever thought that you might be doing something wrong? You can do more harm than good to your face if you are not doing it the right way as it can result in dryness, wrinkles, premature sagging, acne, rashes, irritation and more.

The cleansing procedure will differ for each product range, and it's important to follow the manufacturers' step-by-step instructions on how to apply their products to get the best results. It is crucial to include your neck in your cleansing routine every day, because a lot of people are negligent and when they reach a certain age, they can see a major difference between the face and neck's skin texture. Most of the time it is too late to reverse the signs but it can be improved.

Use a cleanser that will suit your skin type. To keep it simple, choose a cleanser that removes the dirt, germs and excess oil, but still leaves the skin feeling moist and supple afterwards. A harsh unsuitable cleanser will make your skin dry and sensitive, and gives the skin a red undertone.

The best practice is to cleanse your face with lukewarm water temperature in the washbasin, before you take a shower or bath. Removing all make-up, dead skin build-up and environmental debris from the skin, before the pores open due to the hot shower or bath. If pores open with all dirt still on the skin, it seeps deep into the skin, clogging pores.

Another very important fact is that you are not doing your face any favours by cleansing it under the shower. The heat and pressure of the water is in fact causing damage. You cannot cleanse your face under the shower at the same temperature and pressure as what you wash your body. A hot shower can aggravate the fragile capillary networks in the cheeks, leading to unattractive visible capillary networks and worsened impaired skin conditions. In light skin the capillary network directly under the skin surface will be easily noticeable.

After you have cleansed your face and neck with lukewarm water in the washbasin, dry it with a damped face cloth or face sponge which you only use on your face and neck. A facial sponge and cloth has a finer texture than the ones you will use on your body. Keep your cleansing accessories for your face and neck separate from your body's cleansing accessories. This will ensure high hygienic standards, preventing any bacterial infections in the delicate skin of the face and neck. Drying your face and neck with a dampened facial cloth or sponge, will leave a bit of moisture behind to help hydrate the skin. When you use a dry towel to dry the face, you'll dry the skin too much and can leave fluff from the towel behind that can cause irritation.

Your facial cloth or sponge will need regular replacing of around two to three months, or when necessary. The better you look after it, the longer it will last. If you notice any tears, discoloration, and holes, replace the facial sponge immediately, as you may be damaging your skin otherwise with harmful bacteria that may be growing inside the sponge. Never store wet facial sponges in a damp, enclosed place, because it encourages the growth of mould and bacteria. You will notice quickly when you have to replace your facial cloth or sponge. Keep these cleansing accessories hygienic clean at all times to preserve good and young skin. After each use, wash and wring, then hang or place it on a clean spot to dry properly till the next use.

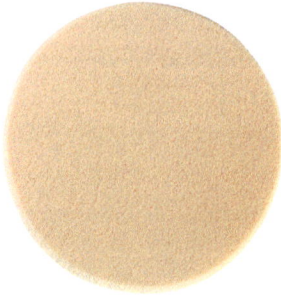

Figure 1

Something that stays wet during the day is a breeding ground for bacteria. You do not want to wash and dry your face and neck with bacteria. The more hygienic your cloths and tools are that you use to keep your face and body clean, the more beautiful skin you'll have.

I use a quality yellow facial sponge for years. It must be a fine textured facial sponge as in figure one that is not harsh to cause any skin damage or sensitivity. This facial sponge is a useful addition to any skin care routine. It helps to draw dead skin, dirt, and cosmetics away from the skin, stimulating the growth of new cells, and even lightly exfoliate the skin preparing it for any special treatment that follows, like a mask or serum. When the dead skin is removed from the surface, skin products that you apply afterwards will be more effective. Yellow compressed facial sponges are hard when dried and must be softened with water first, before using. These sponges are super absorbent and expand on contact with water. That is why it is so efficient when using to cleanse the face and neck, as it absorbs and extracts most of the dirt from the skin.

If you prefer to use a facial cloth, use a soft and fine textured one that is specifically designed for the face. Just as you would use a soft washcloth for a baby, your face and neck requires the same special treatment to preserve it for longer. Exfoliation for the skin is good, but too much and too harsh exfoliating techniques can harm the skin, causing sensitivity. Working too roughly with the skin also causes broken capillaries, called 'spider veins'. They occur when the small veins just beneath the skin's surface dilate, or enlarge.

Tips on how to use a yellow facial sponge for the best results

- When you open the package for the first time, rinse it out several times before using it to ensure that any dust or debris that may have settled into the sponge through the production processed is washed away.

- After each use, wash it with a soft liquid soap to remove any creams and make-up stains. Only soap can remove creams and oil build-up successfully. Rinsing with water alone will leave unwanted oils trapped in the sponge. After washing, rinse a few times under a running tap while squeezing constantly to get rid of all the soap and dirt still trapped in the fibres.

- Place it on a clean block or tray to let it dry completely during the day.

- Before using it again, soften the sponge by submerging it in the clean lukewarm water in the washbasin, wring it and place it on the edge of the washbasin. Wash your face and neck now gently with an emulsion of cleanser and a bit of water. Rinse the face and neck and then use the dampened facial sponge to wipe off the remaining cleanser and water from the face in upwards and sidewards motions. Rinse the sponge a few times if necessary. When done, wash the sponge as already mentioned, and place on a clean block or tray to dry.

- Make sure to clean the block or tray in which the facial sponge gets placed to dry, regularly as well. My suggestion is to clean it every three to four days.

THE DIFFERENT SKIN TYPES

Know what skin type you have, in order to buy the correct skin care products. This piece of information will also help you make the right decision on what skin care routine you'll follow. Skin types usually change with age, and will eventually adjust depending on your diet, lifestyle and hormone balances.

Skin types	Characteristics
1. Young	This is from baby skin to a child aged nine years old.
2. Normal	This is the least problematic skin type because the moisture content of the skin and production of oil are perfectly balanced. There are no dry spots or greasy areas on the skin. It will look clean and clear, and have a healthy complexion.
3. Dry	The most common characteristic of the dry skin is, it's dry and flaky. Skin feels tight and has finer pores with finer lines. Having a dry skin can increase skin irritation.
4. Oily	An oily skin appears greasy and shiny, have enlarged pores, and most likely have pimples, blackheads and/or blemishes.
5. Combination	This is the most common skin type. A combination skin means that you have two different skin types combined. The skin is usually dry to normal on the cheeks and sides of the face, while having an oily skin on the forehead, nose, and chin; called the T-zone. Blackheads and pimples can occur specifically on this T-zone of the face.
6. Problem	A problem skin is a chronic skin condition of some sort. For example acne, rosacea, eczema, psoriasis etc. You cannot use just any skin product for any of these conditions, and will require a specific treatment as prescribed by your GP or dermatologist.
7. Sensitive	The most delicate of all skin types. Skin feels tight and itchy. It is prone to redness, dryness and irritation.

You must take care of your skin and naturally formulated skin products and gentle treatments are recommended. |
| 8. Mature | Skin loses tone and plumpness, wrinkles deepen and the skin looks thinner and drier. This is due to cell renewal that slows down, causing the epidermis to sag. The result is frown lines and crow's feet that settle in, laughter lines appear and liver spots become more apparent. |

THE DIFFERENT FACE AND NECK CLEANSERS

pH Balanced face cleansers come in different forms:

- Liquid (light, medium, heavy)
- Cream
- Soap (liquid, foam, bar)
- Gel
- Facial wipes

Your lifestyle, personality and skin type will determine which cleanser will be best suited for you. For example: If you are a sporty person who exercises regularly or daily, you may prefer a pH-balanced soap or light cleansing milk.

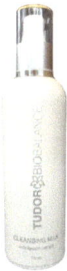

Light liquid cleanser

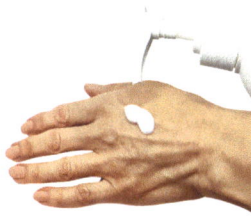

Medium liquid cleanser

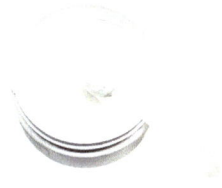

Cream cleanser

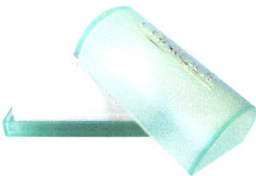

pH balanced bar soap

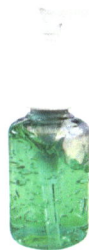

Gel cleanser

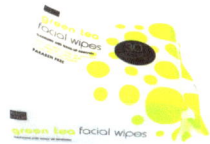

Facial Cleansing wipes

Chart of the different types of cleansers and their uses:

CLEANSER	APPEARANCE	
Liquid a) Light liquid cleanser b) Medium liquid cleanser c) Thick liquid cleanser	a) Oil in water emulsion and is very watery. b) Less watery and a more oily emulsion but still a liquid. c) Thicker emulsion containing more oil than water and is no more a liquid.	
Cream	A thick emulsion which contains oil and is a non-liquid.	
Soap **(pH balanced)**	Soap bars or Liquid soap cleansers like a gel or foam.	
Gel	A gel cleanser does not contain any oil or cream and usually is a clear formula.	
Facial wipes	It is a dampened wipe with the necessary ingredients to clean the different skin types.	

SKIN TYPE	COMMENTS
a) Young and Youthful skin between 6-18 years with perfect skin. Sensitive skin types. b) Youthful skin between 18-25 years or sensitive skin. c) Stronger or dry skin types for people between 25-40 years.	a) Remove all superficial impurities and suitable for teens not wearing make-up. b) Suitable for a person who wears no or little make-up. c) Removes water soluble- and make-up consisting of oils easier.
Dry, sensitive skin and dehydrated or mature skin.	Removes heavier and thicker make-up bases, also lock in moisture for a dry and mature skin.
Oily, Problem and youthful skin with a lot of impurities (for example acne)	a) Must be pH balanced and suit age of the skin. b) Young and mature skin types that produce less oil must use a soap cleanser with an added oil or cream to prevent skin from getting drier over time.
For normal to oily skin types, wearing no or very little make-up.	Gels do not remove thick make-up foundations and creams properly and are best suited for the sporty person or young normal to oily skin who does not wear heavy make-up.
There are different cleansing wipes on the market. Read the label thoroughly and choose wipes best suited for your skin type.	This kind of cleansing is for people on the go. For example: After sport, exercise or gym. It is ideal for people on holiday or when you want to freshen up while flying or camping in the bush. Not recommended to use all the time because it is costly and some may not provide a proper clean every time. It increases the risk of skin pulling & stretching.

The different skin care products and their purpose

Eye make-up remover

Before a woman starts with her face and neck cleansing routine, she needs to remove any lipstick and mascara with eye make-up remover. Apply some eye make-up remover to a dampened cotton round and use gentle circular movements to remove it. The best eye make-up remover consists of one third of oil that will ease the job. Do not work too rough around the eye. Remove the stubborn mascara close to the eyelids by dipping an earbud in lukewarm water and work gently by brushing the eyelashes close to the skin, lifting the tough mascara. Replace with a new earbud if required till all mascara is removed.

Cleanser

The primary function of a cleanser is to remove, sebum and creams successfully from the skin. Make-up bases are oil-based and the only substance to remove them effectively is an oil-based cleanser. The oil emulsifies with the oil in the make-up and lifts it off the skin so that water can wash it away. To get rid of heavy make-up bases, use lukewarm water instead of cold water to wash it away more easily. Milk and cream cleansers are more moisturising and hydrating than soaps, gels and foam cleansers. Your skin type will determine what type of cleanser will work best for you. Dry skin types will benefit from using a cream cleanser that will leave some oil behind to moisturise the skin a bit, whereas soap or foam will be more beneficial for an oily skin to remove all the oil from the skin and give it a matt appearance.

Young and youthful skins usually require a light milk cleanser because the skin has usually a perfect balance of moisture and hydration. The more natural a face cleanser for the particular skin type, the better, so that you do not dramatically change the pH balance of the skin. Some teenagers develop an oily skin and the most likely causes are hormonal changes and overactive sebaceous glands. They will need to use a face cleanser, moisturiser, and mask for an oily skin. Be careful not to use too drying or harsh skin products though, which will dry the skin surface too much, causing the skin to tighten and preventing the trapped oil to escape.

The follicles get blocked by the tightening skin and will form blackheads, whiteheads, and pimples. A teenager must be patient through the years until their skin clears up. Remember that there is no miracle cure for an oily skin. The solution here is to cleanse the face two to three times a day, to keep the oil under control. Teenage girls with and oily skin must stay away from heavy make-up foundations that will form a barrier on the skin, preventing the oil to escape naturally, causing impurities. Another trick is to blot the face a few times during the day with a clean facial tissue to absorb the excess oil. A healthy diet, cutting out too oily and fatty foods will limit the oil produced by the skin.

Toner

This is an important part of any skin care routine. It's usually a watery product with added active ingredients that you apply to a dampened cotton round, and then gently blotting or wiping over the face and neck after you have cleansed the skin with a cleanser. A good toner will remove any remaining bits of oil, dirt and debris left behind after cleansing. More importantly, a toner will help soothe, nourish and hydrate the skin while restoring its delicate pH balance. A toner that has vitamins and antioxidants will help refresh the skin, providing a boost of energy and calming effect. Ingredients such as aloe vera, or witch hazel will naturally tighten the skin to improve the overall look. Stay away from a toner that has added alcohol to it, as it will dry the surface of the skin too much. Even if you have a very oily skin it is not good to dry the surface of the skin while the oil is still trapped under the skin, finding it hard to escape. The toner can have a slight natural tightening effect to close the pores after cleansing, but not an extreme drying effect.

Exfoliator

This removes dead skin cells from the surface or outer layer of the skin, creating a smoother appearance and stimulating the production of new skin cells. The exfoliator cream has added microbeads to help with a gentle scrubbing effect. By removing the build-up of dead skin and creams on the skin, also enhances the skin's ability to absorb special ingredients or medications you apply afterwards. These microbeads must not have sharp edges that will easily cut or damage the skin. The amount of exfoliating treatments per week will depend on the skin type. For example: An oily to problem skin will exfoliate twice a week, whereas a sensitive skin may only exfoliate once a week, or even once every second week. Do not use a body exfoliator on the face and neck, as it is usually too harsh for the delicate skin of the face. Use an exfoliator specifically manufactured for the face and neck containing gentler microbeads.

Moisturiser

Moisturising your skin every day can help keep your skin clear, smooth, and wrinkle-free for longer. The correct moisturiser for your skin type will reduce skin problems. By applying a moisturiser to a dry skin will add the needed moisture and help keep its pH balance through the day. Using a foam or soap cleanser on the oily skin will remove the unwanted layer of oil on the skin surface, and help keep the pH balance better during the day. By removing the extra oil produced on the skin will eliminate bacterial working on the skin. Applying a moisturiser to your face can increase the moisture level of the outermost layer of the skin, preventing it from drying out.

A moisturiser for a dry and sensitive skin has more of an oil ingredient in, to form a protective layer on the skin surface, preventing more drying of the skin. Where a moisturiser for the oily skin type will have less of an oil base, and more of a moisturising base, to add the needed moisture to the skin. It is not uncommon for an oily skin to be dehydrated. The excess oil produced by the skin may camouflage the fact that the skin lacks moisture. A person with an oily skin will do their skin the world of good by drinking six to eight glasses of water per day, to hydrate the skin from within. Moisturisers containing a SPF (sun protective factor), will protect the skin against sun damage, and minimising pigmentation or age spots forming due to ultraviolet light exposure by the sun.

Night Cream

A night cream is much richer in texture and is formulated to use at night. They aren't absorbed by the skin as quickly as most moisturisers and lotions. It can double the skin's moisture content and support anti-aging benefits. The skin types that will benefit most by using a night cream at night are the mature, dry, and sensitive skins.

Special treatments for the skin include

Masks
Facial masks treat a particular skin type or condition. There are many different face masks and depending on each mask's properties, they can help hydrate the skin, remove excess oils, improve the appearance of the pores, heal, calm, soothe, rejuvenate, or just simply pull out impurities. A face mask is a special treatment for the skin and must not be overused. When used too many times during a week, they can in fact have a negative impact. Use a mask according to its instructions, and as a rule, not more than twice a week with enough days of rest in between. A facial mask is applied after cleansing, exfoliation and extractions, and before the toner and moisturiser.

Masks come in different formulas such as clay masks, peel-off masks, cream masks, thermal masks, warm-oil masks and natural masks. Oily and problem skin types will benefit more from applying a clay, peel-off, or natural mask, to remove the oil and impurities from the skin. Dry, normal, and mature skin types will use a mask that add more moisture and oil to the skin, rather than stripping away the oil and moisture content. Sensitive skin types will use natural based mask formulas that will cause minimal to no irritation.

Make sure to use the correct mask for your skin type and problem, otherwise you'll create more problems for the skin than solving it. Scoop the right amount of mask from the pot with a spatula or teaspoon, and then apply it evenly with clean fingers or a mask brush to the face. You can include your neck as well. Follow the instructions of the specific product carefully. When removing a clay mask, always use a yellow face sponge and clean lukewarm water to moisten the dried mask on the skin first. Use gentle wiping movements, without pulling and stretching of the skin. Rinse the facial sponge a few times during the removing stage. Remember to thoroughly clean the sponge with a liquid soap afterwards to remove any remaining mask from the fibres of the sponge.

Serums

A serum is a concentrated treatment for the skin. The most common benefits include hydration, increased nourishment, strengthening of skin cells, cell renewal, brightening of the skin, wrinkle improvement, reducing the size of the pores, and the prevention of acne. While face creams contain around 5 to 10 per cent of active ingredients, a face serum can contain up to 70 per cent. Serums are made up of smaller molecules that can penetrate deeper into the skin, to deliver a very high concentration of active ingredients. They are the first products that should be applied to the skin after cleansing and toning, before applying the moisturiser and make-up.

Other special treatments to reverse skin damage

These are treatments that are ministered by a professional beauty therapist or physician to give the skin a more youthful appearance. Skin peels, laser treatments, non-surgical anti-ageing treatments, skin needling. If you want to know more, visit a qualified beauty therapist to find out the best treatment for your desired results.

I personally use the *Tudor BioBalance* from Australia that is a beauty salon quality skin product range with natural ingredients, and no chemicals to harm the skin in the long run. Choose your skin product range carefully by firstly looking at the ingredients and their benefits. Secondly, test it on your skin for at least seven days and monitor how your skin reacts throughout. How does your skin feel after applying it? The skin must not feel dry, irritated, or oily. It must have a supple look to it. Check with the supplier if they can provide you with enough testers to last a week. Some suppliers sell travel kits that work well so that you do not have to buy the full quantity, until you are sure it is working well for your skin. Especially when the cost is pricier than the products you can buy from pharmacy stores.

Be careful of the following: When you have to keep using a certain skin product, to see good results on your skin. There are a lot of moisturisers and skin products that have seen the light over the past few years creating outstanding results, connected to 'build your own business' through multi-level marketing. Women pay good money for these lotions because they see immediate results in looking younger. What they do not realise, is that most of these lotions consist of toxic ingredients that irritate the skin, making it swell due to the inflammation it creates. As the skin swells, the body sends water to the area to try and wash the toxin away and the wrinkles look softer. Some fine wrinkles even disappear. Toxic ingredients will over time exhaust your skin and make it sag more, because it lost its natural reproductive elements. You are at risk of premature aging if you use toxic chemicals continuously on your skin.

THE DO'S AND DON'TS OF SKIN CARE

Do's

- Cleanse and moisturise the skin twice daily - morning and night.

- Apply a moisturiser with a SPF during the day to protect against harsh sun rays.

- Use a cleanser that will suit your skin type i.e. young, normal, dry, oily, etc.

- Always use a pH balanced face cleanser.

- Wash your face in the washbasin first with lukewarm water, before you take a shower or bath.

- Include your neck in your daily cleansing routine.

Don'ts

- Do not wash your face under the shower. The water temperature is too warm.

- Do not use normal hand soap to wash your face, as it is not pH balanced.

- Do not work rough when cleansing and moisturising the skin.

- Do not use chemical based skin products that will do more damage over time. Stick with natural and clean ingredient products.

FACE CLEANSING STEPS FOR TEENAGED GIRLS AND WOMEN

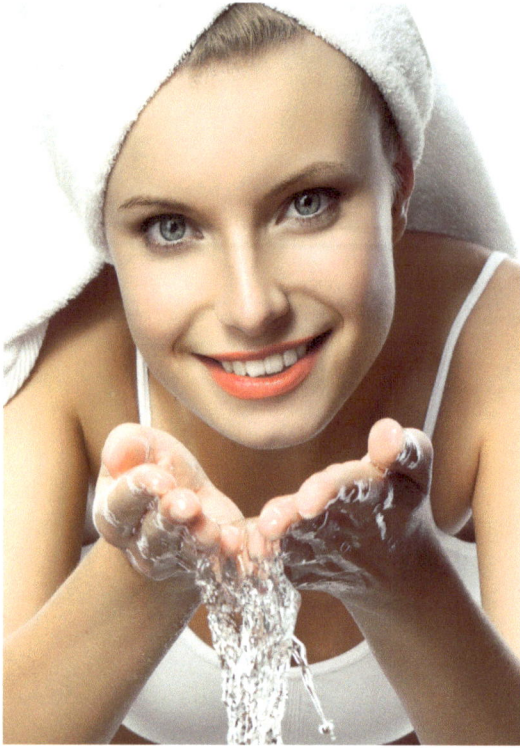

Teenaged girls will use light and natural products as their skin is still young and supple. Heavy cleansers and creams can cause irritation.

Apply a light sunscreen over the moisturiser every day, to preserve young skin for longer. Because they are still very active, they must avoid heavy make-up bases and foundations that will prevent the skin from breathing easily during the day, causing clogged pores and skin breakouts.

We all have different skin types, and therefore we should use skin care products for our specific skin. If you are not sure what skin type you have, you can always ask a beauty therapist to perform a skin analysis on you.

The following face cleansing steps should take a woman between two-three minutes in the morning and night (excluding the mask and exfoliator):

Step one:

Wash your hands first. This is an important step that most people ignore. It is important to wash your hands first because cleansing your face with dirty hands means you are transferring all the dirt and germs on your hands, onto your face.

Step two:

Eye make-up and lipstick removal. Use two dampened round cotton pads to applying the eye make-up remover. Wetting the cotton round and squeezing most of the water out, will spare your product over time. When you pour the eye make-up remover on a dry cotton pad it will suck up too much of the product. A good eye make-up remover will remove the eye make-up and mascara quickly, without having to use harsh rubbing or pressure. A hybrid of water and oil is the best eye make-up remover. The oil helps to break down the make-up, and lifts it off the skin and eyelashes quicker.

Hold the first cotton pad on a closed eyelid for about five-ten seconds before starting to remove the eye shadow and mascara in a couple of gentle circular motions. Clean gently because the skin texture around the eyes is delicate. If you are working too roughly, you can stretch the skin and over time you'll produce more or deeper wrinkles.

To remove the remaining mascara successfully from the eyelashes close to the skin, use earbuds dipped in lukewarm water, and gently clean between the eyelashes as close as you can to the eyelid.

Use the second dampened cotton pad with eye make-up remover to remove any lipstick on your lips.

Step three:

Cleanse the face and neck by using a cleanser and normal to luke-warm water temperature. A low water temperature will keep your skin hydrated and unaffected. Avoid using too warm or too cold water to wash your face. Too warm water washes away essential oils from the skin, leaving it dry. The skin of our face will become too dry, and may even produce aggravation or outbreaks. Whereas using very cold water irritates the skin, causing broken capillaries which are tiny veins visible near the surface of the skin. Skin pores cannot withstand extreme temperatures.

Before hopping in the bath or shower, fill the washbasin with luke-warm water. Rinse your face with the water first to give it a wet base to work with. Pour a small amount of face cleanser in one hand, add a bit of water, and rub quickly between the hands to spread the cleanser, transfer the cleanser on your hands with a swift circle motion over the whole face and neck, now start cleansing your face with your fingers for 30 seconds to one minute in gentle circular motions. Dip your fingers in the water if the cleanser on the face is too dry and hard to spread. Then rinse your face with the water in the basin to remove most of the cleanser.

Wipe your face clean with a soft, clean and dampened face cloth or yellow face sponge. It's not that easy to rinse the neck though, and is best to gently wipe it clean with the soft face cloth or sponge in upwards motions. Rinse the cloth or sponge a couple of times during the time otherwise you'll just move the cleanser on the neck from one spot to another.

Afterwards, wash the washcloth or face sponge with a bit of baby shampoo or liquid hand soap to remove any mascara or make-up that got trapped in the fibres. Make sure to rinse the face cloth or sponge thoroughly to get rid of any soap and hang the face cloth, or leave the face sponge to dry on a clean tray.

Women who apply loads of make-up during the day will find that when cleansing the face, the oil and waxes form a dirt line in the washba-sin. Out of courtesy for the next person who wants to use the washbasin, do not forget to clean it quickly with a soft nail brush and liquid hand soap while pulling out the basin plug.

Step four: (Include this step only once or twice per week)

- **Gentle exfoliating of the skin.** An exfoliator removes dead skin and increases blood circulation, resulting in a rosy glow. Do not use too frequently and choose an exfoliator that is not harsh causing damage to your skin. Avoid the delicate area surrounding the eyes. Never use an exfoliator more than three times a week. Overusing an exfoliator can disrupt the natural skin barrier and can cause dryness, irritation, and excess oil production. Fill the washbasin three quarters with lukewarm water. Rinse your face with the water first, pour a dime sized amount of exfoliator in one hand, use two fingers of the other hand to spread it all over the face. Gently massage the product all over the face for about 30-45 seconds. Focus on areas where dead skin and build up primarily occur like the nose, forehead, chin and neck.

- Remove the exfoliator completely from the skin with your face cloth or face sponge before you apply the mask.

- **Apply a special facemask once to twice a week after you have exfoliated the skin.** Exfoliating prepares the skin to absorb more of the active ingredients in the mask. If your skin produces breakouts after using a mask two times a week, change the schedule to only once a week. Rinse and remove the mask completely from your face after the leave-on time. Leaving some residues on the face can clog the pores and dry the skin later. Rinse thoroughly especially at the hairline, neck and sides of the nose. These are the places often missed and can lead to skin irritation later.

- For a mask that hardens, you'll have to wet it all over the skin with a wet face cloth or face sponge to soften the mask, before removing it gently. Do not rush to remove a hardened mask because you will use unnecessary pulling and stretching on the skin. Take your time and rinse the face cloth or sponge a few times to remove the mask successfully. Wash the face cloth or sponge with a liquid soap under a running tap to rinse away any remaining mask trapped in the fibres. You may want to cleanse your face again with the face cleanser before you move on to the toning step.

- Always wipe your face with a clean and dampened face cloth or yellow face sponge after the product was removed from the skin. Avoid using the towel kept close to the washbasin since it is used by everyone in the family, and it carries a lot of germs that will end up on your skin. If you are using a face cloth, do not rub the skin dry, instead just pat it dry. When you are using a yellow face sponge to dry the skin, use light strokes. Leaving a fine mist of water on the face, will help seal the moisture into the surface of the skin when you apply a moisturiser or cream over it.

(Shower or bath now before continuing with steps five-seven)

Step five:

Wipe the skin with a toning lotion. Use a dampened round cotton pad and pour or spray the right amount of toner on it. Now wipe the skin gently to remove the last traces of cleanser or mask from the skin. A toner will prepare your skin for the moisturising step.

Step six:

Apply eye cream. Don't be as heavy-handed with your eye cream as you would with your moisturiser. Dab the eye cream in with sideways motions along the bottom and top eyelids. Avoid applying it too close to the eyes, which will cause irritation or sensitivity. Use your ring finger to do this because the muscles in this finger are generally weaker, so they're not likely to pull too much on this delicate area that will cause irritation or wear and tear on the skin.

Ensure to apply the eye cream at the right stage of your skincare routine. The aim is to get all skin care products to absorb properly into the skin. The rule of thumb is to apply your skin care lotions and creams from the lightest product to the heaviest, this way the heavier products can penetrate through the lighter ones. So if your eye cream is richer and denser than your moisturiser, apply it after the moisturiser. If it's lighter than your moisturiser, apply it before, and continue with this rule. Any serums that are lighter than both the eye cream and moisturiser should be applied first.

Step seven:

Lastly, apply your moisturiser or cream. Apply a moisturiser immediately after cleansing your face while the skin is still damp. Waiting until your skin is completely dry makes it harder for the active ingredients to get properly absorbed into the skin, and cause the skin to feel greasy or tacky.

FACE CLEANSING STEPS FOR TEENAGED BOYS AND MEN

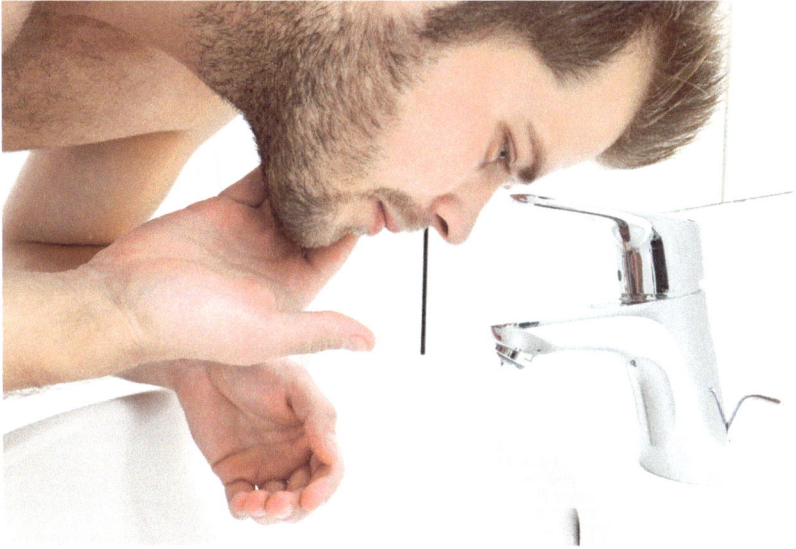

Facial care for men is just as important and it isn't just a woman's practice. Real men also do facials. There's nothing vain or feminine about it. A guy with a solid, energised face gets noticed. Men's skin care at home can be straightforward and easy. There is no need for five-step peels or multiple layers of creams. A simple daily routine with good quality skin care products will do the trick. It is also very important to cleanse the face morning and night. Men with beards and moustaches must clean all the exposed skin. Wash your beard and moustache with a beard shampoo one to two times a week. Avoid using normal hair shampoos as it is too harsh for the delicate skin of the face.

Teenaged boys should also use age-appropriate products which are light and natural. Wearing a moisturiser with a sunscreen in direct sunlight is a must to preserve young skin for longer. Men in the trade profession and working in the sun regularly must take special care to protect their exposed skin with a sunscreen, clothing and hat. A greasy type of sunscreen can discourage men from applying it daily, therefore I would suggest buying a non-greasy or light feel sunscreen and moisturiser. This will keep you in the habit of applying it every day. A good quality pair of sunglasses is beneficial to protect your eyes against the harsh sunrays. Wearing the right shape of sunglasses frame that fits your face shape, will make you look cool!

The below face cleansing steps should take you only two-three minutes (excluding the mask and exfoliator):

Step one:

Wash your hands first. Cleansing your face with dirty hands means you are transferring all the dirt and germs, or grease on your hands, onto your face.

Step two:

Cleanse the face and neck with a men's face wash or cleanser in normal to lukewarm water temperature. A low water temperature will keep your skin hydrated and unaffected. Avoid using too warm or too cold water to wash your face. Too warm water washes away essential oils from the skin, leaving it dry. Whereas using very cold water irritates the skin and causes broken capillaries underneath the skin. Cleanse your face separate from your bath or shower routine because the water temperature that we bath and shower with is too warm for our face. The skin of our face will become too dry, and may even produce aggravation or outbreaks. Your skin pores cannot withstand extreme temperatures.

Before hopping into the bath or shower, fill the washbasin with lukewarm water. Rinse your face with the water first to give it a wet base to work with. Pour a small amount of face cleanser in one hand, add a bit of water with the other hand, and rub quickly between the hands to spread the cleanser, transfer the cleanser on your hands with a swift circle motion over the whole face and neck, now start cleansing your face with your fingers for 30 seconds to one minute in gentle circular motions. Dip your fingers in the water to add water to the cleanser on your face if it is too dry and hard to spread. Then rinse your face with the water in the basin to remove most of the cleanser. Wipe your face clean with a soft, clean and dampened face cloth or yellow face sponge. It's not that easy to rinse the neck, and is best to gently wipe it clean with the soft face cloth or sponge in upwards motions. Rinse the cloth or sponge a couple of times during the time otherwise you'll just move the cleanser on the neck from one spot to another.

Afterwards, wash the washcloth or face sponge with a bit of baby shampoo or liquid hand soap to remove any grease or dirt trapped in the fibres. Make sure to rinse the face cloth or sponge thoroughly to get rid of any soap and hang the face cloth to dry, or leave the face sponge to dry on a clean tray.

Oils and creams on the face will form a dirt line in the washbasin. Out of courtesy for the next person who wants to use the washbasin, do not forget to clean it quickly with a soft nail brush and liquid hand soap while pulling out the basin plug.

Step three: (Include this step only once or twice per week)

- **Gentle exfoliating of the skin.** An exfoliator removes dead skin and increases blood circulation. Men are strong and therefore must be careful not to scrub the skin too hard and roughly with the exfoliator that has beads in, because you can cut and damage the skin. Fill the washbasin three quarters with lukewarm water. Rinse your face with the water first, pour a dime sized amount of exfoliator in one hand, use two fingers of the other hand to spread it all over the face. Gently massage the product all over the face for about 30-45 seconds. Focus on areas where dead skin and build up primarily occur like the nose, forehead, chin and neck. Avoid the delicate area surrounding the eyes. Never use an exfoliator more than three times a week. Over-exfoliating can cause dryness, irritation, and excess oil production. When you are done with the exfoliating process, rinse off with lukewarm water. Pat your face dry with a clean face towel/cloth.

- **Apply a special face mask once to twice a week after you have exfoliated the skin.** A lot of men do not particularly like to apply a mask and wait for 10-15 minutes before removing it. If you are one of those men, my suggestion is to apply a mask that stays moist just

41

before you get into the shower. So when you get out of the shower and has dried your whole body, five minutes would have passed, then you can remove the mask. You need the mask on your face for at least five minutes for the active ingredients to have any impact on the skin. If this whole skin cleansing routine is all new to you, and you do not feel comfortable with all the fuss, just skip the mask step for now until you are more comfortable to add it to your skin routine later. By cleansing your face and neck the correct way is a huge improvement already, and you can be proud of yourself!

- When your skin produces breakouts after using a mask two times a week, change the schedule to only once a week, or you may even have to change to a different mask that is not that rich for your skin type. Follow the instructions of the product on how long you need to keep it on the skin before removing it. Rinse and remove the mask completely from your face. Leaving some residues on the face can clog the pores and dry the skin later. Rinse thoroughly especially at the hairline, neck and sides of the nose. These are the places often missed and can lead to skin irritation later.

- For a mask that hardens, you'll have to wet it all over the skin with the face cloth or sponge to soften the mask, before removing it gently at the end. Do not rush to remove a hardened mask because you will use unnecessary pulling and stretching on the skin. Take your time and rinse the face cloth or -sponge a few times to remove the mask successfully. You may want to cleanse your face again with the face cleanser to remove the last traces of the mask, before moving on to the next step.

- Always wash the face cloth or sponge with a liquid soap under a running tap to rinse away any remaining mask trapped in the fibres. I recommend that men do not use a hardened mask unless they have an oily skin type. Hardened masks take time to remove which men do not particularly like. Use a mask that stays moist or creamy, and are mostly feeding the skin.

Step four:

Shaving the skin. (See how your skin is doing when shaving straight after the exfoliating or mask. If your skin is too sensitive to shave then wait till after you have showered or bathed before continuing with shaving). After exfoliating and mask, shave your face with a sharp razor to eliminate any sensitive skin, and then rinse with lukewarm water. Pat your face dry with a clean face towel. A tip to keep your razor sharp for longer and rust free: after each use, dry it with a towel and store it in a dry place like the bathroom cabinet, till the next use. Alternatively shave in the morning, then exfoliate and apply your mask at night, on the days you have allocated for these special treatments.

(Shower or bath now before continuing with steps five-seven)

Step five:

Apply a toner. Men may ask: 'What is a toner?' Well a toner may be the missing link that a men's skin care regime has been crying out for. Toner is designed to remove the excess oil that causes 'shine', preventing the pores from becoming clogged with creams and cleansers (causing blackheads), it helps eliminate or control breakouts, refresh your complexion, sooth the skin after shaving, and prevents irritation. Use a toner that is alcohol free though, because alcohol will dry the skin too much, and have a burning sensation on the skin after you have shaved. Apply an alcohol free toner to a dampened cotton pad, and use gentle sweeping or dabbing motions on the skin in the direction of hair growth so that the cotton do not stick to any stubble.

Step six:

Apply your eye cream. Don't be heavy-handed and only use a very small amount. Use your ring fingers, which are generally weaker so they're not likely to pull or rub on this delicate area. Dab the eye cream in with sideways motions along the bottom and top eyelids. Avoid applying it too close to the eyes which will cause irritation or sensitivity.

Step seven:

Apply a moisturiser to your face which includes a SPF (Sun Protective Factor) of at least 15 SPF in the mornings. You only need a little bit of product and there's no need to vigorously rub it in. Pat it in across the whole face and neck. It is recommended to use a higher SPF (30 or 50 SPF) when you are working in direct sunlight for longer than 30 minutes. Re-apply the SPF 30 or 50 after four hours when working for longer periods in the sun. Use a normal night cream or lotion at night. Even a light day cream or lotion will work at night which does not include a SPF. For the dry and mature skin a cream or thicker lotion will help lock the moisture in the skin.

Remember to use a body lotion for your arms and hands every day as well. You do not want to keep your face and neck younger for longer, and then the skin on your arms and hands give away your real age.

Congratulations if you follow this skin routine! I know it will pay off and your skin will stay younger for longer.

FACE CLEANSING STEPS FOR GIRLS AND BOYS UNDER THE AGE OF TEN

General advice and good practices to teach children under the age of ten are as follows

When your child is a baby and toddler, it is easy as mum and dad will be bathing them with baby soap that is usually soft and pH balanced. By the time they get to the age of six, mum and dad normally leave them to become a bit more independent when it comes to washing and bathing themselves. Teach them the following: They shouldn't stretch their skin through the cleansing procedure, or in general. Cleanse their face in lukewarm water before taking their bath. They are very young and will not be able to successfully cleanse their neck separately, therefore it is important to buy a pH balanced soap to wash their neck with the rest of their body when bathing. Make them aware how important it is to rinse all the soap or cleanser from their face before taking a bath. This will get them in the right routine for the rest of their life. They do not wash their face again while bathing.

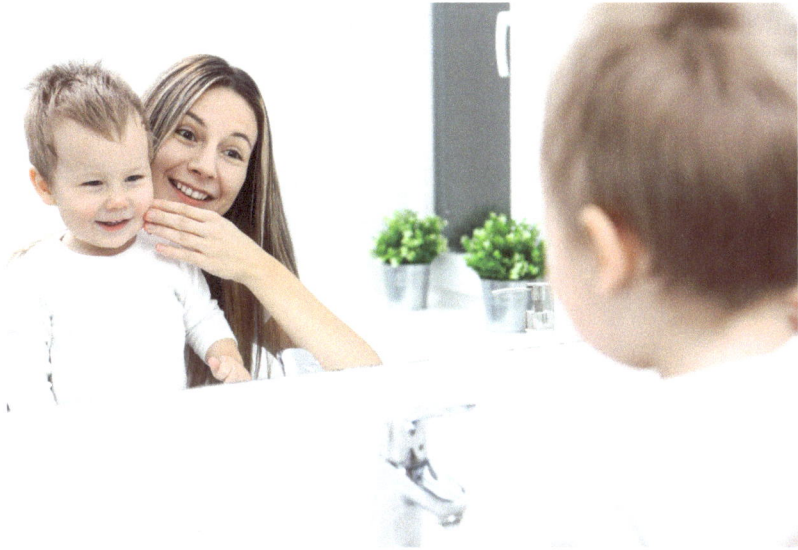

After their bath, dry their body and apply a moisturiser or skin lotion that is age-appropriate and light for their skin. I recommend that they have two washcloths, one for their body and one for their face that is softer in texture to prevent any rough working to the delicate skin of the face. A washcloth suitable for babies is ideal for their face. Teach your boy and/or girl that it is crucial to wash and rinse their washcloth after each use, wring it well, and hang it to dry. This will eliminate bacterial growth in the fibres. Mum or dad can even throw all family members' washcloths in with the weekly towel wash load to help keep them clean, and last for longer.

Obviously children will not use expensive, heavy cleansers and moisturisers that are formulated for the adult skin. Some active ingredients that are found in lotions and creams meant for the adult skin, can cause sensitivity or even harm their beautiful young skin. A light baby skin lotion will work well at night time. In the morning they must apply something that is light but also have a SPF (Sun Protective Factor) of at least fifteen. Buy a non-greasy moisturiser for them as an oily appearance does not look good and will annoy them during the day.

Children must be educated how delicate the skin around their eyes is, and they'll need to take special care to work very gentle around their eyes. It is not good to rub the eyes with their hands as it will become a habit, and continuous rubbing will cause wrinkles sooner as they are getting older. Show them how to use only the right amount of product so that they are not wasting unnecessary amounts.

Children between six to nine do not need to use special treatments like masks or exfoliating but will benefit from natural feeding masks every now and then for example: blending cucumber with other natural ingredients like honey or yogurt serves as a refreshing face mask for your child's skin. A thin layer of mashed avocado is rich in Vitamins A, B1, B2, D, E and other essential oils, and works well for dry and sensitive skin. There is no need to apply it for longer than five minutes though and remember to wash their face before applying this natural mask.

The below steps are for children aged 6-9 and should take them only one-two minutes (excluding the natural face mask which is optional):

Step one:

Wash their hands first. They must wash their hands first, not to transfer any dirt or germs from the hands onto their face.

Step two:

Cleanse the face with a pH balanced soap or liquid cleanser in normal to lukewarm water temperature. Wash their face before they bath. Fill the washbasin half to three quarters with lukewarm water. Splash the face with water first, then wash the face with the pH balanced baby soap or liquid cleanser. When they use a facial soap, lather the hands with the soap and bit of water. Now wash the face for 5-10 seconds by lightly rubbing in circular motions.

After the face was cleansed, rinse the face to remove most of the cleanser. Use a soft dampened face cloth to gently wipe the face clean. Wash the face cloth quickly with the liquid hand soap, thoroughly rinse all the soap out, then wring and hang up to dry for the next use.

Now bath before continuing with step three. Do not wash the face again when showering or bathing. After you have towel dried and dressed, continue with the next steps.

Step three: (optional)

Every second week to a month they can apply a natural food mask for five minutes at this stage. When the natural face mask is successfully removed, move on to the next step. Some children love the pampering with mum or dad when they do their face routine, and some don't. Do not force your child if they do not like putting on a mask.

Step four:

Apply a small amount of baby face lotion on the face and neck. Apply a body lotion that is chemical and fragrance free on the arms and legs to combat any dry and itchy skin. To protect their delicate face and neck during the day when they are out in the sun to play, apply an oil-free moisturiser or sunscreen of at least 15 SPF(Sun Protective Factor) in the mornings. If they are out to play for longer periods cover more exposed skin with a SPF lotion. As it is important that children get a short burst of sun early in the morning or late in the afternoon to help with the production of Vitamin D, there is no need to always cover them up with sunscreen. Judge when the intensity of the sun is high to protect their skin.

THE IDEAL SKIN CARE ROUTINE FOR WOMEN AND MEN IN A WEEKLY TABLE:

Day	Steps for morning procedure	Steps for night procedure
Sunday	1. Cleansing 2. Skin toner 3. Eye cream 4. Moisturiser with a SPF*	1. Cleansing 2. **Gentle exfoliating** 3. **Mask** 4. Skin Toner 5. Eye cream 6. Moisturiser / night cream
Monday	1. Cleansing 2. Skin Toner 3. Eye cream 4. Moisturiser with a SPF*	1. Cleansing 2. Skin Toner 3. Eye cream 4. Moisturiser / night cream
Tuesday	1. Cleansing 2. Skin Toner 3. Eye cream 4. Moisturiser with a SPF*	1. Cleansing 2. Skin Toner 3. Eye cream 4. Moisturiser / night cream
Wednesday	1. Cleansing 2. Skin Toner 3. Eye cream 4. Moisturiser with a SPF*	1. Cleansing 2. **Gentle Exfoliating** 3. **Mask** 4. Skin Toner 5. Eye cream 6. Moisturiser / night cream
Thursday	1. Cleansing 2. Skin Toner 3. Eye cream 4. Moisturiser with a SPF*	1. Cleansing 2. Skin Toner 3. Eye cream 4. Moisturiser / night cream
Friday	1. Cleansing 2. Skin toner 3. Eye cream 4. Moisturiser with a SPF*	1. Cleansing 2. Skin Toner 3. Eye cream 4. Moisturiser / night cream
Saturday	1. Cleansing 2. Skin Toner 3. Eye cream 4. Moisturiser with a SPF*	1. Cleansing 2. Skin Toner 3. Eye cream 4. Moisturiser / night cream

* SPF – Sun Protective Factor

If the days for the exfoliator and mask in the above table do not work for you, move it to a more suitable day to fit in your weekly life schedule.

THE EFFECTS OF THE SUN ON THE SKIN

The human skin needs sunlight to help produce vitamin D, which is necessary for normal bone formation. Too much sunlight on the other hand will damage or kill skin cells. Skin damage is determined by the extensity and the quantity of sunrays. If you want to stay healthy and look younger for longer in life, you must protect your skin from too much sun. Get your recommended dose of sun every day for optimum health, but know at what time of the day is the safest. Exposure to excess sun causes most of the wrinkles and age spots on our faces. In most cases sun damage to the skin cannot be reversed, but it can be improved at any stage of your life.

Although many people still think a tan looks healthy, it is actually a sign of DNA damage. The skin darkens in an imperfect attempt to prevent further injury, which can lead to the cell mutations that trigger skin cancer. Regular tanning also causes premature aging of the skin and could make you look years older than you actually are. Too much sun exposure over years can make you look 10-15 years older when you get to your fifties and sixties.

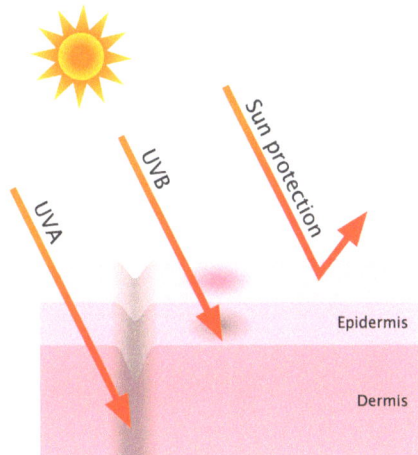

The sun radiates three different sunrays, ultraviolet A (UVA), ultraviolet B (UVB), and ultraviolet C (UVC).

UVA rays are long enough to reach the skin's dermis layer, damaging collagen and elastic tissue. Recent studies show that UVA might have contributed to certain cancers. UVA rays are also used in tanning booths.

UVB rays are the main cause of reddening and sunburn. They tend to damage the epidermis, or outermost layer of the skin, where the most common forms of skin cancers occur.

UVC rays are the strongest and most deadliest of solar rays, however luckily for us, the ozone layer stops these from reaching the earth.

The Skin Cancer Foundation says that exactly what kinds of damage UVA and UVB causes to the skin, and how best to protect ourselves, seems to shift every year as new research comes out. For example, it was once thought that only UVB was of concern, but we keep learning more and more about the damage caused by UVA. And new, improved forms of protection against UVA keep emerging. Keeping up with these new developments is a worthwhile challenge that can help all of us preventing sun damage. Both UVA and UVB penetrate the atmosphere and play an important role in conditions such as premature skin aging, eye damage (including cataracts), and skin cancers.

UVA rays are present with relatively equal intensity during all daylight hours throughout the year, and can penetrate clouds and glass. They penetrates the skin more deeply than UVB, and have long been known to play a major part in skin aging and wrinkling, but until recently scientists believed they did not cause significant damage in areas of the epidermis (outermost skin layer), where most skin cancers occur. Studies over the past two decades have shown that UVA damages skin cells called keratinocytes in the basal layer of the epidermis, where most skin cancers occur. Therefore UVA contributes to and may even initiate the development of skin cancers.

Frequent and prolonged exposure to UVB rays over many years is the main cause of the most common skin cancers. Another type of skin cancer called Melanoma, is thought to be caused by brief, intense exposures, such as a blistering sunburn. UVB also contributes to skin aging. Its intensity varies by season, location, and time of day.

Examine your skin often for suspicious growths or changes in an existing skin lesion. Early detection and treatment is the key to the cure of skin cancer. Remember to cover up with a sun protective factor (SPF) when you are going to be in harsh sun for longer than five minutes. SPF is a relative measure of how long a sunscreen will protect you from UVB rays.

HOW TO PROTECT YOURSELF FROM DAMAGING SUN RAYS

The best sunscreen to use is a broad spectrum sunscreen that protects against UVB and UVA rays. There is no sunscreen that can block sunrays a hundred per cent and you will have to take caution not to stay in the sun for too long. The time that you can stay safely in the sun is different for every skin type and skin colour, and is also determined by the sun protective factor (SPF) number of the sunscreen.

HOW MUCH DO THE DIFFERENT SPFs BLOCK UVB RAYS?

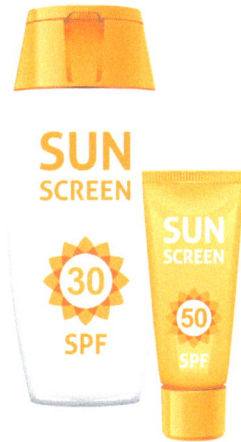

SPF 15 blocks 93% of UVB rays.
SPF 30 blocks 97% of UVB rays.
SPF 50 blocks 98% of UVB rays.
SPF 100 blocks 99% of UVB Rays.

Ultrahigh SPFs does not protect more than the SPFs 30 or 50. To work out for how long you can sit in the sun for, with the different SPF factors, use the following equation:

MINUTES YOU BURN WITHOUT SUNSCREEN X SPF NUMBER
= MAXIMUM SUN EXPOSURE TIME

For example: If you take 10 minutes to burn work it out as follows:

10 minutes X 15 SPF = 150 minutes (two hours 30 minutes)

This is the time you can stay in the sun for, but you also must take in consideration the intensity of the sun on a particular day and time.

The skin makes most Vitamin D when it's exposed to the midday summer sun, and that's the time the skin is most easily damaged. In warmer countries located in Africa, South America and Australia where the sun comes through very strong, you'll need to protect your skin from the sun between 10am-3pm. Sometimes even earlier or later, depending on the intensity of the sun and season. Therefore it is safer to sit in the sun before or after these times to get your recommended sun exposure for optimum vitamin D production. Low vitamin D levels can cause osteoporosis, a condition in which bones lose calcium, become brittle and are susceptible to fracture.

People with very dark skin need around six times more exposure to UV radiation to produce as much vitamin D as a person with fair skin. Fortunately they are less likely to get skin damage because of greater amounts of pigment in the skin, protecting from the sun.

Recommended sun exposure times for the different skins for optimum production of Vitamin D are as follows.

Fair skin: 5-10 minutes in summer, and 7-30 minutes in winter.

Darker skin: 15-60 minutes in summer, and 20 minutes to 3 hours in winter.

It is important to also take in account the latitude and intensity of the sunrays. When you experience a sting in the skin from the sun, move to the shade. Exposure to the arms is all you need to get your recommended dose of sun per day.

HYGIENIC PRACTICES FOR COSMETICS AND SKIN PRODUCTS

Correct hygiene practices are essential to maintain good and healthy skin. Apply your moisturiser and a cream with clean hands. Keep your facecloths and sponges clean. Avoid sharing facial creams and skin products with others. If you have to share, use a small spatula so that each person can scoop out just the right amount for each use. Sharing products with others can result in product wastage when everyone does not know how much to scoop each time. Don't share towels or personal washcloths and sponges either.

Do not at any time dip your fingers straight into your cream pots, use a clean spatula or plastic tea spoon to scoop out the right amount of product. Our hands are considered to be the most unhygienic part of the body, because we have to touch everything during the day. Cross-contamination will occur in our creams if we just dip our fingers straight in it. Microbes can grow almost anywhere. These tiny organisms bring with them some distasteful product changes or even disease. Alternatively, opt for products that come in tubes or have an airless pump. You can even buy your own airless pump and transfer your favourite jar products hygienically.

Scooping too much product is a waste of money, and in some instances can do more harm than good to your skin when you over apply. Never place any remaining product on the spatula back into the jar, in the case where you have scooped too much. It is better to scoop just a small amount at first, because you can always scoop a bit more if needed. After you have scooped out the cream, wash the spatula or spoon and store in a clean/dry container for the next use. Remember to clean the container regularly as well.

Thoroughly close the jars, tubes and bottles after each use to avoid prolonged contact between skin products and the air. From time to time it is recommended to clean the edge of jars, tubes and caps, and remove any creams that remain on them with a clean facial tissue. Bacteria and fungi that grow in skin products may cause various unpleasant skin reactions, and they thrive in warm and humid conditions. That's why cosmetics and skin products should be stored in a cool, dry place away from direct sunlight. Please note that products quickly deteriorate when they come in contact with heat and stored in extended warm conditions. You can store creams and lotions in the refrigerator if the environment you live in is too warm. The ideal temperature is 8-12 degrees Celsius or

46.4-53.6 Fahrenheit. They are no use to you if the product properties changed because it will not do the job it was created for. Also remember to watch out for expiration dates.

What is a skin product's expiration date? The printed expiration date on the label of each skin care product indicates the guaranteed effectiveness of the active ingredients within the product. After this expiration date the product has lost its effectiveness.

By law, manufacturing companies must show the expiration date and/or the production date, as well as the 'product after opening' symbol on the packaging.

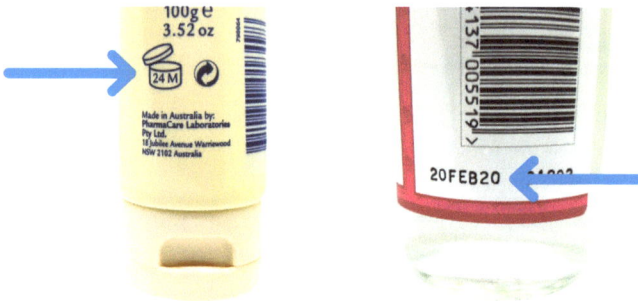

Meaning of production date, expiration date and PAO

Production date or manufacture date is the date when the product was manufactured. More precisely, it is the date when the batch of cosmetics or skin products was produced. This date can be printed on the package, but also can be omitted.

Expiration date is the date after which the products will be expired and should not be used anymore. Usually this date must be specified only for products which shelf life period is 30 months or less. If this date is present, it should be printed directly on product packaging in the form of month/year or day/month/year, for example: Exp. 09/24 means that you can use the product only till the end of September, 2024; Exp. 15/06/2024 means that the product can be used only before the15 of June, 2024.

When the shelf life of the product is more than 30 months (e.g. 3 years), the expiry date will probably not be printed. But this doesn't mean that you can use the product during the whole 3 years or more. You'll then have to look at the PAO symbol.

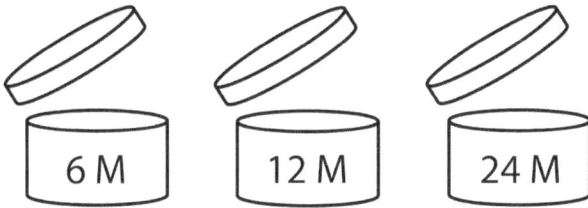

Examples of PAO Symbols

Period after opening (PAO) symbol is to clarify how long you can use the product for once you have opened it. Find the 'open jar' symbol at the bottom/back of the packaging. There will be a number followed by the letter 'M'. The 'M' stands for months and the number in front of it indicates for how many months the product can be safely used for, after you have opened it. For example, 6M means that the product can be used for six months after opening, 12M means twelve months and 24M means twenty four months etc.

Generally speaking, you can keep your cosmetics *unopened* for up to three years after production date. This is a general term, and can depend on the product and company who produced it. As soon as you opened it, you should maintain the PAO date. Organic cosmetics usually do not include preservatives, and can be stored only for up to 6 months after opening. A tip is to label the products with the first date of use, so you know when it is time to replace it.

The red flag must be when you notice any changes in your creams and cosmetics. This can mean that the shelf life has come to an end, or bacterial invasion is to blame. Changes can come in the form of bad smell, discolouration, change in consistency, or the obvious growth of mould in the product.

It is very easy to determine mascara that expired, as soon as it is dry, throw it away. Do not try and revive it by adding water. Mascara as a rule only lasts for three months. That is why big brand cosmetic companies produce small tubes. Nail polish can be considered worthless when it began to thicken and harden. If you have any suspicion about the appearance or odour of a product, it is better not to use it anymore. Skin care products that are off can cause very nasty effects on the skin. Some effects can take months to heal and others can be irreversible.

SIMPLE HOME REMEDIES FOR THE FACE AND NECK

As already mentioned, it is better to use skin care products that are free from chemicals. To protect your skin from any harm or damage by those harmful chemicals, what better way than to use homemade beauty remedies that you can make from natural foods and ingredients? Keep in mind that an individual with a problem skin must consult their general practitioner or dermatologist first, before using any of the below remedies. Although natural products usually cannot do any harm, it may clash with any form of medicated creams that you already use.

REMEDIES FOR GLOWING SKIN

Remedy One

For normal/dry/ combination/mature/ sensitive skin.

(If there is any reaction or itchiness when using this on the sensitive skin, stop using it immediately)

Ingredients: 1 tbsp. virgin coconut oil

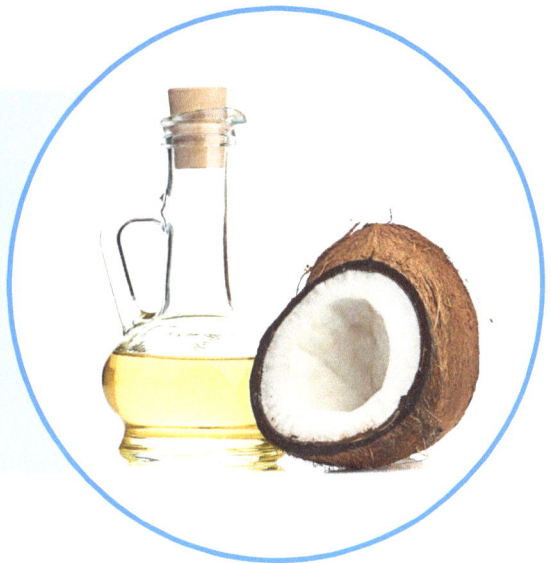

Method:

1. Melt hardened coconut oil on a low heat or place it in a small stainless steel bowl over hot water so that it is easy to apply to a clean face and neck and after your shower at night. Be careful not to apply hot or too warm oil to the face. Let it cool down first.

2. Now massage the skin with gentle circular motions for a couple of minutes. Do not pull the skin down, but rather use upwards circular motions.

3. Leave the oil on overnight, but if it is too oily, blot it with a clean facial tissue. Not toilet paper as the fluff can cause skin irritation. Wash it off in the morning with your face cleanser.

* You can use coconut oil on the skin every night, or as often as you want.

This remedy works best for dry and dull skin. Coconut oil locks the moisture in the skin and also nourishes it with essential fatty acids. Its phenolic compounds contribute to its antioxidant activity and give you glowing skin.

Remedy Two

For all skin types (individuals with problem skin must check with their dermatologist first)

Ingredients: 1 tbsp. aloe vera gel, 1 t. honey, 1 t. milk, a pinch of turmeric.

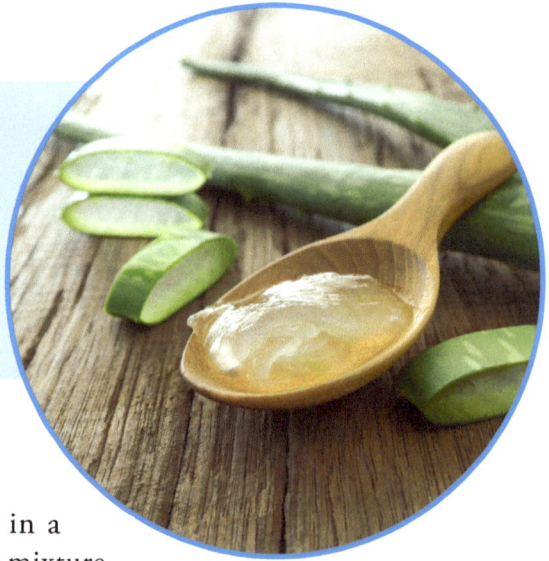

Method:

1. Mix all the ingredients in a small bowl and apply the mixture evenly to a clean face and neck.

2. Leave it on for 20 minutes.

3. Rinse off with lukewarm water.

4. Wipe skin dry with a damp yellow face sponge.

* Apply this face mask up to twice a week.

Aloe vera gel is the ultimate solution for skin problems. Its nourishing and healing properties rejuvenate the skin to give it a natural glow. Turmeric has healing power and also contributes to a natural glow. Honey is naturally antibacterial, and full of antioxidants which are great for slowing down aging. Milk has a calming and nourishing effect on the skin.

Remedy Three

For all skin types (for individuals with problem skin check with your dermatologist first)

Ingredients: 1 t. baking soda, 1t. extra virgin olive oil, ½t. honey.

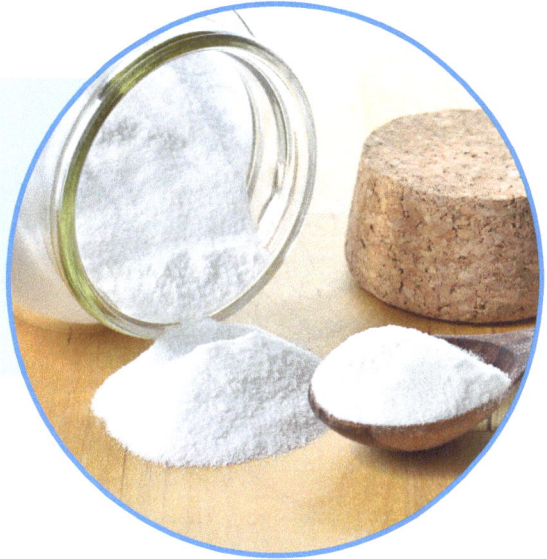

Method:

1. Mix all the ingredients in a small bowl.

2. Apply the mixture on a clean damp face and neck using circular motions. Avoid the skin directly around the eyes.

3. Leave it on for ten minutes.

4. Rinse off with lukewarm water and wipe skin dry with a damp yellow face sponge.

5. Wipe the skin clean with a toner, then apply your eye cream and moisturiser as usual.

* Apply this face mask once a week.

Baking soda exfoliates dead skin cells and also neutralises the skin's pH. It soothes the skin and heals any inflammation that may be present as well. Combined with honey that is an antioxidant, and extra virgin coconut oil that moisturises, it will give you glowing skin.

Remedy Four

For all skin types
(Individuals with problem
skin must check with their
dermatologist first)

Ingredients: 1 t. Honey

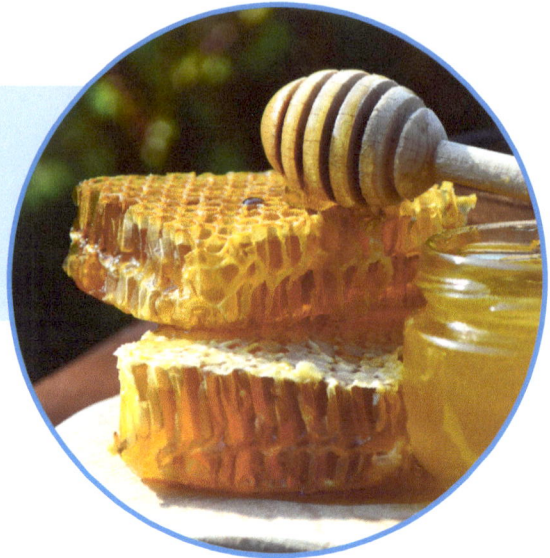

Method:

1. Apply honey evenly on clean and damp skin.

2. Massage the honey for a few minutes and leave it on for another five minutes.

3. Wash off with lukewarm water and wipe skin dry with a damp yellow face sponge.

4. Apply your toner, eye cream and moisturiser as normal.

* You can apply a thin layer of honey 2-3 times a week.

Honey has antimicrobial properties that clean and make your skin soft. It is also rich in antioxidants, reducing blemishes and ensuring a healthy skin.

Remedy Five

For normal/dry/
combination/mature and
sensitive skin.

(If there is any reaction
or itchiness when using
on the sensitive skin, stop
using it immediately)

Ingredients: 1 tbsp. olive
oil, a small clean soft
towel, bowl with warm
water.

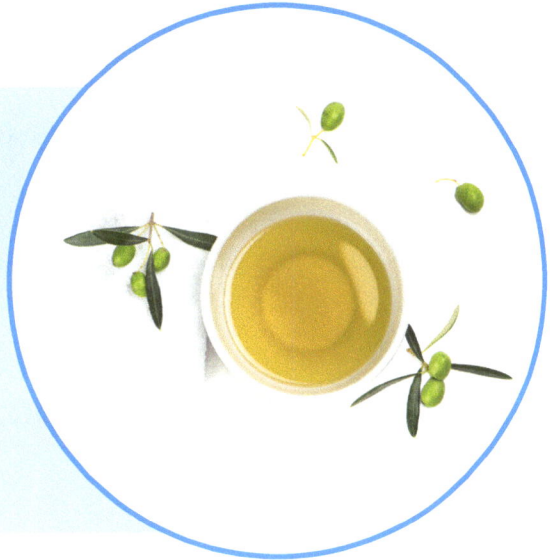

Method:

1. Apply a few drops of oil on your fingertips, and apply it all over a clean face and neck.

2. Massage in upward circle motions for 2-3 minutes, especially on your cheeks, nose, and forehead.

3. Dip the towel in the warm water, wring out the excess water, and place the towel on the face for 30-40 seconds, while lying on the bed relaxing. Leave your nose open for breathing.

4. Dip the towel again in the warm water, wring out excess water, and gently wipe away the oil on the skin.

5. Pat your skin dry with a facial tissue if required.

* You can use olive oil and a warm towel on the skin every night, or as often as you want.

Olive oil is an excellent skin moisturiser and provides a natural shine to the skin. The flavonoids and polyphenols present in olive oil protect the skin from free radicals and prevent damage. It repairs the skin cells and makes it healthy and glowing.

NOTE: DO NOT OVERUSE MASKS ON THE FACE AS IT CAN OVER-FEED OR OVER-STIMULATE, CAUSING BREAKOUTS ON THE SKIN. USE A MASK MAXIMUM TWICE A WEEK. REFER TO THE 'THE IDEAL SKIN CARE ROUTINE IN A WEEK TABLE' AT THE END OF 'CLEANSING YOUR FACE THE CORRECT WAY' SECTION. USING TWO DIFFERENT MASKS PER WEEK, TREATING TWO DIFFERENT PROBLEMS ARE ALLOWED.

Remedy Six

For normal/dry/combination/mature and sensitive skin.

(If there is any reaction or itchiness when using on the sensitive skin, stop using it immediately)

Ingredients: One ripe banana, 2 teaspoons milk.

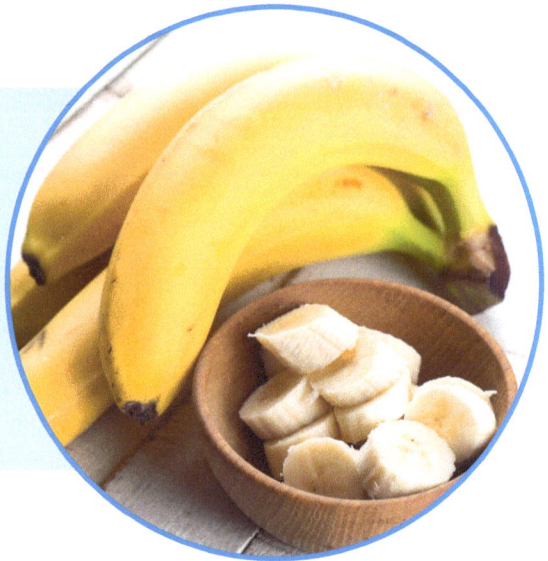

Method:

1. Mash the banana in the milk and apply it on a clean face and neck.

2. Leave it on for 15 minutes.

3. Rinse off with lukewarm water, and wipe skin dry with a damp yellow face sponge.

4. Apply rosewater or toner to a damp cotton round, and wipe lightly or dap all over the face.

5. Apply your eye cream and moisturiser as usual.

* Apply this banana mask on your face once or twice a week. If your skin breakout after using this mask it is too rich for your skin type. Cut down on the times you apply, or cut out completely.

Banana is rich in Vitamins A, B, C, and E, and minerals such as potassium that nourishes and hydrates the skin. It makes the skin soft and glowing, but also lightens blemishes.

Remedy Seven

For all skin types.

Ingredients: Rose water, 1 x cotton ball or cotton round, small bowl.

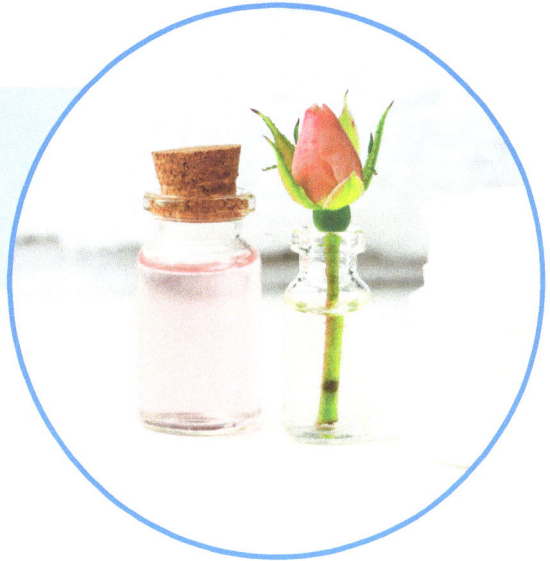

Method:

1. Cleanse the face and neck first with a pH balanced facial cleanser or natural cleanser.

2. Pour two tablespoons of rosewater in a small bowl and dip the cotton ball or round in the rose water, squeeze out excess rose water but still wet enough.

3. Apply it all over your clean face and neck.

4. Dip in the rose water again when the cotton becomes dry.

5. Apply your eye cream and moisturiser as usual.

* You can apply rosewater to the face and neck every morning and evening after you have cleansed the face, before applying your moisturiser or cream.

Rose water is commonly used as a skin toner to cleanse and refresh the skin. It improves the skin tone by stimulating blood circulation and balances the pH of the skin.

REMEDIES TO CLEAR UP A SKIN FROM ANY BREAKOUTS

Remedy Eight

For oily/problem/and combination skin types.

Ingredients: 2 tbsp. of finely chopped fresh mint leaves, 2 tbsp. natural yogurt, 2 tbsp. oatmeal.

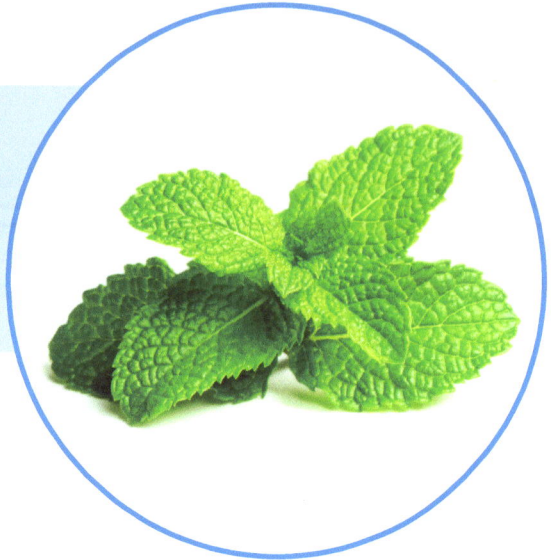

Method:

1. Mix all the ingredients in a blender.

2. Apply to a clean face and leave on for 10 minutes. For the combination skin, only apply the mask on the T-zone (oily forehead, nose and chin).

3. Rinse off with lukewarm water and wipe skin dry with a damp yellow face sponge.

4. Apply rosewater or toner to a damp cotton round, and wipe lightly or dap all over the face.

5. Apply your eye cream and moisturiser as usual.

* Apply this mint mask on your face once or twice a week.

Mint can help clear blocked pores from oil and clear acne before it begins. The lactic acid present in the yogurt will help hydrate the skin. Oatmeal has anti-inflammatory properties.

Remedy Nine

For oily/problem and combination skin types.

Ingredients: One green tea bag, or 3-6 green tea leaves, or one teaspoon of dried green tea leaves, Cotton ball or cotton round.

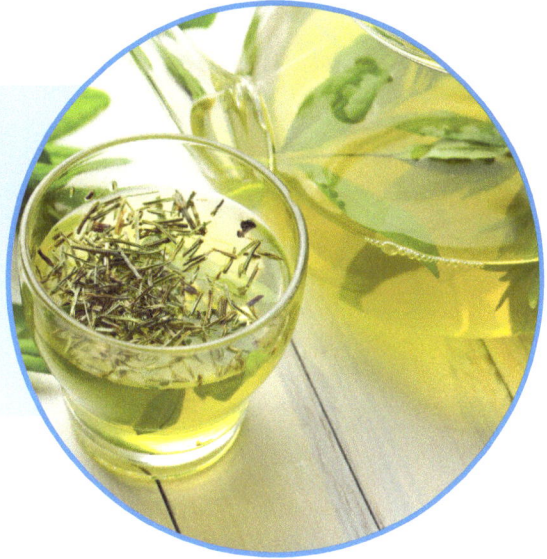

Method:

1. Brew the tea for five-ten minutes and let it cool down.

2. Cleanse the skin with your normal face cleanser and wipe skin dry with a damp yellow face sponge.

3. Dip the cotton ball or round in the green tea, and squeeze out the excess green tea water so that it is just damp. Put this cotton now on the side to use after you have rinsed the face with green tea.

4. Rinse the face a few times with the green tea water, then wipe the skin dry with the dampened green tea cotton that you have put on the side.

5. Wait five minutes for the green tea to be fully absorbed by the skin before applying your eye cream and moisturiser.

* Use this remedy once to twice a week.

Green tea has antimicrobial and antioxidant compounds that can help fight breakouts on an oily and acne skin. It may shrink enlarged pores and the antioxidant present in green tea can fight against the signs of aging. Any person with a problem skin that is under medication or medicated creams must check with their dermatologist first if this remedy can be used with their medication.

Remedy Ten

Natural eye make-up removers for all skin types.

Ingredients: Use any one of the following natural oils on a dampened cotton round. Coconut oil, olive oil, jojoba oil, almond oil.

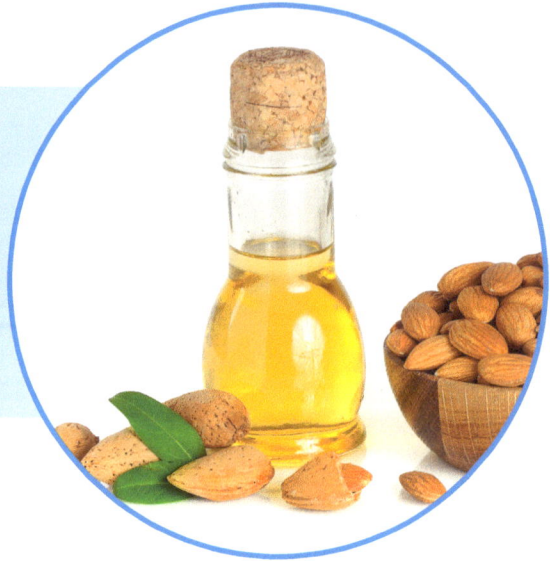

Method:

1. Dip a cotton round in water and squeeze the excess water out.

2. Pour a bit of your chosen natural oil on the damped cotton round.

3. Gently remove your eye make-up.

4. For stubborn mascara, dip an earbud in warm water and remove mascara by working the earbud between the eyelashes close to the skin.

5. Remove the remaining oil gently from the eye area with a lukewarm damp cotton round and rose water.

* This remedy can be used every day.

These natural oils are gentle and will remove the eye make-up easier and quicker without you having to work too rough around the eye area. Just be careful not to let the oil come into the eyes.

FACIAL REJUVENATION TREATMENTS

It is hard for a lot of people to accept the aging process of the body, especially in their face. That is why facial rejuvenation is a multi-billion dollar industry every year where some people would do whatever possible to keep their youthful look. This is especially the case where skin damage is so far that you'll require some extra help to improve it. An unfortunate situation arises when a person overuse these facial rejuvenation procedures to the point where they do not look like themselves anymore. They get so addicted to these procedures that their appearance starts to look unnatural or in worse cases, malformed. The purpose of this section is to explain to you that there are other procedures available to help improve your skin's appearance, but also informing you to be careful not to go overboard. When a person has gone too far, there is nothing that can be done to reverse some procedures. Trying to fix mistakes will just make it worse every time.

I do not see a problem if someone wants to take that extra step in improving their appearance, but rather would encourage you to use all the tips and advice already mentioned in this book, to help you age gracefully in a more natural way. When you look after your skin properly, you'll require minimal to no permanent facial rejuvenation procedures, to have an attractive appearance. One thing that all of us on this earth cannot escape from is to go through the normal aging process. The only control we have over the aging process is to slow it down by looking after our skin, eating healthy foods, and to work regular exercise in for the improvement of bodily health. Our aim must be to have an attractive appearance all the way as we ages, and not to stay young forever.

Trying to stay young forever will look unnatural and will make you feel unhappy, as it is impossible to look like your best youthful years forever.

Facial rejuvenation is a cosmetic treatment, or series of cosmetic treatments, which aims to restore a youthful appearance to the human face. It can be achieved through either surgical or non-surgical procedures.

Surgical facial rejuvenation procedures can include a brow lift or forehead lift, eye lift, facelift, chin lift and neck lift. *Non-surgical* facial rejuvenation treatments can include, but is not limited to chemical peels, wrinkle relaxers (such as Botox®), dermal fillers, laser resurfacing, photo rejuvenation, radiofrequency and ultrasound.

Cosmetic surgery: Cosmetic surgery focuses on enhancing a person's appearance. It is elective and focuses on the aesthetics of beauty. Cosmetic surgery procedures include:

- Breast enhancement: Augmentation, lift, reduction.
- Facial contouring: Rhinoplasty, chin, or cheek enhancement.
- Facial rejuvenation: Facelift, eyelid lift, neck lift, brow lift.
- Body contouring: Tummy tuck, liposuction, gynecomastia treatment.
- Skin rejuvenation: Laser resurfacing, Botox® injections, filler treatments.

Plastic surgery: Focuses on repairing defects to reconstruct a normal function and appearance. Plastic surgery is defined as a surgical specialty dedicated to reconstruction of facial and body defects due to birth disorders, trauma, burns, and disease. It is intended to correct dysfunctional areas of the body and is reconstructive in nature. Examples of plastic surgery procedures are:

- Breast reconstruction.
- Burn repair surgery.
- Congenital defect repair: Cleft palate, extremity defect repair.
- Lower extremity reconstruction.
- Hand surgery.
- Scar revision surgery.

Chemical peels: This is a technique where a chemical solution is applied to the skin, like a mask that causes the skin to 'blister' and eventually peel off. The new skin is usually smoother and less wrinkled than the old skin.

Wrinkle relaxers: Are used to rejuvenate the face and reduce signs of ageing that comes in the form of injections or creams. The most effective form of relaxing the muscles is still injections, because it will relax the muscles for a few months. Whereas a relaxing cream is only a temporary solution that may cost more over time. Most of you reading this book would have heard the word Botox. It is the trade name for a wrinkle relaxer injected into the skin, known to inhibit muscle movement and prevent further wrinkle developing or wrinkle worsening.

Botox®, also called Botulinum Toxin, and is made from the bacteria that cause botulism. Botulinum toxin blocks nerve activity in the muscles. It also treats severe spasms in the neck muscles, muscle spasms or stiffness, certain eye muscle conditions, overactive bladder and incontinence, multiple sclerosis, the prevention of chronic migraine headaches in adults, even treating severe underarm sweating.

The effects from Botox® on the face will last anything from three to six months. As muscle action gradually returns, the lines and wrinkles begin to reappear and need to be treated again. When you want to look good for an event, you'll have to get Botox® injections ten to fourteen days before the event, as it takes a bit longer to work through the muscles to produce a smoother or wrinkle-free look. Botox® does weaken the muscles, and the more you get an anti-wrinkle relaxer, the fewer units you'll need when you continuing on a three to six month schedule, as the muscles weaken. Another effect of constantly weakening the muscles for many years is that skin sagging will be more visible when you stop receiving anti-wrinkle relaxer injections. The simple explanation is that muscles that do not get regular exercising will shrink and waste away, known as atrophy. Muscle tissue will decrease in bulk and length, resulting in a noticeable loss of size and definition. This is not extremely bad, as the face is not a body part like the arm or leg that needs to be strong to help you work and move.

There is no specified age for getting Botox®. Young adults in their early twenties get it as a preventative measure to stop wrinkles from forming, and weaken the muscles not to repeatedly move more times than necessary, which again will stop the forming of new wrinkles. Botox® does not get rid of all wrinkles on your face, but only the ones made by facial expressions. It does not get rid of what we call static wrinkles, or the ones that are seen when at rest.

Botox® injections have minimal side effects when done by an experienced injector, but there are long term risks and damages recorded.

Always ask your chosen injector of the risks beforehand, also ensure he or she has the experience and a good track record.

Dermal fillers: Are a non-invasive treatment used to restore youth and volume to the face. Restoring volume and plumpness to lips, chin, cheeks, the jawline, the area under the eyes, and even the nose. Fillers can also be used to improve the appearance of scars. Dermal filler injections are quick and provide instant results with a minimal amount of discomfort or downtime. Depending on the type of filler, the effects can last anywhere from six months to two years. Dermal fillers are used to correct signs of aging that are beyond what skin care products can do. The procedure involves injecting a gel substance under the skin that plumps out grooves.

Fillers are divided into two main groups: Temporary fillers that are made from hyaluronic acid that eventually gets absorbed into the body. More permanent fillers are made from materials that can remain in the body for many years.

Thinking of getting dermal filler injected? Make sure to go to a professional that knows what they are doing. There is no 'reversing of the filler' if the injector makes a mistake, or if there is a miscommunication of what you're wanting from your facial filler injections. Top cosmetic injectors insist on using only temporary dermal fillers for your facial injections, rather than a more permanent solution lasting for years. Temporary fillers are better than permanent fillers because they can be adjusted to the face that still ages every day or to your personal preferences over time. The right amount of plumpness for more youthful lips in a woman in her early forties may simply look over done and 'overly enhanced' five years later.

Douglas McGeorge, a consultant plastic surgeon and president of the British Association of Aesthetic Plastic Surgeons, said: 'The public needs to be realistic about the outcomes it can expect from new cosmetic treatments, at least until solid clinical evidence of their efficacy exists'. He added that failure to bring in statutory regulation of people offering such treatments would lead to serious health problems in the future. 'To foster a wild-west approach of industry self-regulation is not only an affront to reputable professionals who follow the rules, but ultimately creates an unsafe environment for the public'. His warning was echoed by other plastic surgeons who are warning that long-term use could permanently damage skin.

I have included a section on facial exercises later in this book, which can be used as an alternative in ensuring firmer skin. Just as any muscle in the body needs exercise to give it a beautiful firm form, the facial muscles needs exercise as well. But there is the right way to do facial exercises, and a wrong way. Read more about this further on.

Laser resurfacing: Is a treatment to reduce facial wrinkles and skin irregularities, such as blemishes or acne scars. Consult a plastic surgeon or dermatologist to find out if you're a good candidate. Laser resurfacing of the skin may be an effective long-lasting wrinkle treatment, but there may be drawbacks for some. A study shown laser resurfacing using a carbon dioxide laser, reduced the appearance of wrinkles by forty five per cent more for two years after treatment. Researchers say carbon dioxide lasers work by vaporizing water molecules inside and outside cells, which damages the surrounding tissue. The skin's natural response to this damage is to produce more of the protein collagen, reducing the appearance of wrinkles.

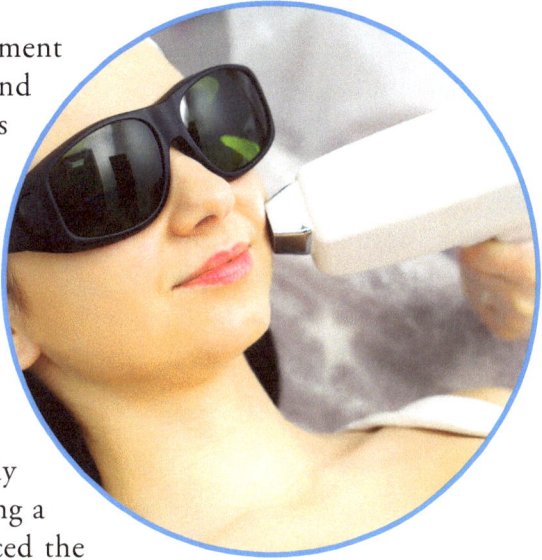

Photo rejuvenation: This is a skin treatment that uses lasers, intense pulsed light, or photodynamic therapy to treat skin conditions and remove effects of photo aging such as wrinkles, spots, and textures. The process induces controlled wounds on the skin, prompting it to heal itself by creating new cells. This process reverses the signs of photo aging to a certain extent by removing appearances of damage. The term 'laser' originated as an acronym for 'light amplification by stimulated emission of radiation'.

Radio frequency: It is an aesthetic technology that uses radiofrequency energy to heat tissue and stimulate subdermal collagen production to tighten the early signs of loose or sagging skin. Typically, treatment requires a series of 8-12 treatment sessions lasting for 30–45 minutes. The process also requires extreme care in its execution because improper application may result in dents on the skin surface due to uneven healing responses on the skin. Therefore make sure you get this treatment to be administered by a qualified professional.

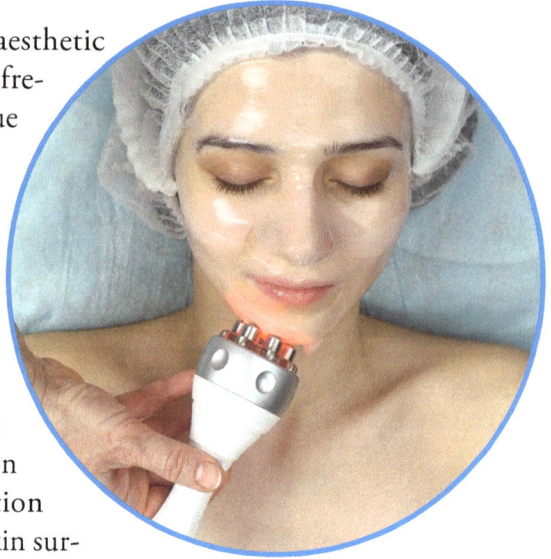

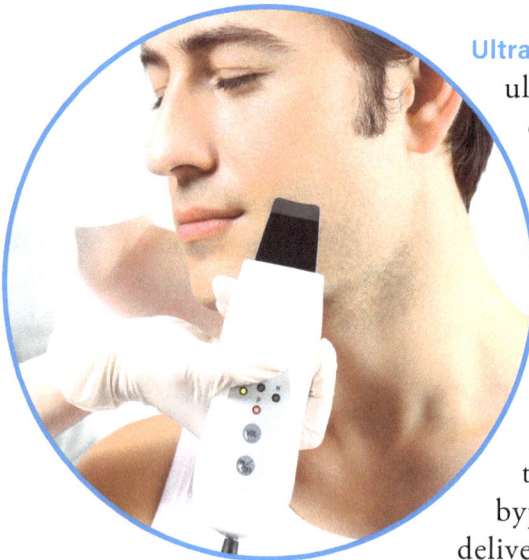

Ultrasound: Practitioners use the ultrasound therapy to target deep tissue layers. They can use the device to focus energy where it is most needed. Non-invasive ultrasound energy is used to lift the skin of eyebrows, neck and under-chin. Unlike other laser treatments that simply target the outer layers of the skin, ultrasound therapy bypasses the skin's surface. It delivers the collagen stimulating ultrasound energy to the deepest layers. The ultrasound skin tightening device reaches five millimetres deep under the skin, penetrating into the second layer of muscles underneath the facial muscles. Lasers don't even go that deep. Ultrasound therapy is a good alternative for those who do not want a face-lift.

IMPORTANT ADVICE FOR COSMETIC CORRECTIVE PROCEDURES

Don't forget, as with any cosmetic corrective procedure, you still need to use well-formulated skin care products and sun protection as part of the anti-aging treatment that will keep your skin looking younger and healthier for longer.

My advice to every person who is thinking to undergo cosmetic surgery is not to solely look at the cost of the procedure, but the quality of the service and the experience of the surgeon or practitioner that you are going to use. There are too many sad stories out there where people went for the cheapest option and ended up malformed, or scarred for life. Do not jump straight into a decision and make sure you do your research on what can be expected from going through a specific procedure. If you are going to spend quite a bit of money, it is best to get it done properly and by an expert, than running the risk of being on the list of surgical mistakes.

The worst decision that you can make is to go through any cosmetic surgical procedure because someone is pressuring you. For example, when your friend our spouse wants you to do it for their own selfish reasons. It's a big mistake wanting to improve your appearance merely for someone else. Your decision must be based on what you want, doing it for yourself. People need to be content with who they are, and love themselves. We are all born with certain features making us unique. By trying to look like someone else is going to be disastrous in the first place, and secondly, may make you even unhappy in yourself afterwards.

Most of the time it turns out that rather than changing something drastically like going through permanent cosmetic surgery, a person only needed a new hairstyle, new wardrobe, and caring for their skin, hands and feet; to feel like a new person. So think really hard about what it is you really want to achieve, before going through with permanent changes which you may regret later. My philosophy is not to perform any permanent changes to my body that cannot be reversed.

People's values and mindset also transition around every five years. So what you think you want today will not be the same you would want in five to ten years' time. But you can never go wrong with treatments that will improve the skin's appearance like laser resurfacing, photo rejuvenation, radio frequency, or ultrasound therapy. The only thing you need to worry about here is choosing the practitioner or beauty clinic with care.

BUILDING BLOCKS FOR GOOD AND HEALTHY SKIN

Just as it is important of what you use on the skin topically, even more important is what you do from the inside of the body to nourish the skin. It is hard to get rid of skin problems on the outside, when the inside keeps producing the problem. That is why I want to touch briefly on how we have to look at what we eat, drink, and do with our body.

THE BASIC BUILDING BLOCKS OF A GOOD AND HEALTHY SKIN

Eating a healthy diet every day. The following foods can be eaten and seen as healthy foods: fresh fish, avocados, all green leaves and salads, cold pressed extra virgin olive oil, green tea, nuts (including walnuts, almonds, cashew, pecan, macadamia, pistachio, hazelnuts), grass-fed beef, organic chicken, organic or pastured eggs, pumpkin, carrots, oranges, fresh berries (like blue berries, mulberries, raspberries, strawberries), watermelon, apples, almond milk, grass-fed butter, other organic fruits, broccoli, cauliflower, cabbage, onions, garlic, ginger, cinnamon, honey, herbs and spices, a small piece of 70% plus dark chocolate per day, one cup of coffee or herbal tea a day without sugar and milk (adding a teaspoon of honey and almond or coconut milk will be okay). True organic produce are the best to eat, and will benefit your body the most.

Drink 6-8 glasses of clean or filtered water per day. Drinking enough water every day will keep your skin looking good and stay younger for longer. Our body is composed of about 60 per cent water and requires enough water per day to maintain the balance of bodily fluids. Water energizes the muscles and controls calories. The kidneys do an amazing job of cleansing and getting rid of toxins in the body, as long as we intake adequate fluids. Water also helps with healthy and normal bowel function every day, preventing constipation and bloating. Eliminate or minimise sugary drinks and alcohol to the bare-minimum. If you are not used to drink that much water a day, start with a glass a day for the first week, then increase to two glasses per day the next week, continue increasing until you reach the requirement amount. Our body also needs to adjust to the water intake. Drinking too much water too soon can make you feel sick, it will then be easy to stop and fall back into old habits again.

Daily exercise and/or movement of the body. Not sure if you feel like I do sometimes? When I am at home for a few days and do not walk or move enough during the day, I start to get aches and pains all over my body. Failure to get enough oxygen to your muscle tissues from lack of exercise can create muscle soreness. When your tissues do not get enough oxygen, lactic acid is created for use instead. Too much lactic acid in your tissues then causes trigger points to form, and is associated with increased muscle tension. If you experience muscle tension from lack of exercise, it's important not to jump back into exercise aggressively either. You should slowly add low-impact exercises like walking or cycling for short bursts of time into your routine. Increase the intensity of exercise slowly so that your body adjust at an acceptable rate.

Having enough rest per day. Depending on your age and circumstances, get six-eight hours of uninterrupted sleep every night. The quantity of your sleep is important, but it's the quality of your sleep that you really have to pay attention to. Some people may sleep for nine hours a night but don't feel well rested when they wake up, because the quality of their sleep is poor. The quality of your sleep does not only affect your physical health, but also your mental state. Getting enough quality sleep every day will produce good skin, a healthy immune system, a good emotional state, contribute to a healthy brain and heart, help with better concentration during the day, keep your weight in balance, and even allow your brain to come up with new creative ideas and inventions to change the world!

Keep a positive attitude every day and avoid stressful situations. Our body is designed to experience stress and react to it. Positive stress keeps you alert and ready to avoid danger. Negative stress is when a person faces continuous challenges without relief or relaxation between challenges. When stress becomes greater than our ability to cope, it can affect our quality of life and cause problems with physical and mental health. Stress affects every person differently and it is important to know how it affects you.

Notice the early signs and deal with it before it becomes a problem. Identify your triggers. A situation that causes one person to become over-stressed may not be a problem for another. A small amount of stress can be a good thing and increase energy and motivation. Stress that continues without relief can lead to a condition called *distress* that is a negative stress reaction. Positive thinking helps with stress management and can even improve your health. Stop negative self-talk to reduce stress. Removing anything negative, whether it's a habit or even a loved one from your life, is very crucial to living a positive life. When you are positive, you are happy. Early warning signs to identify stress: headaches, muscle tension, poor sleep and insomnia, irritability, low energy, chest pain, rapid heartbeat, cold or sweaty hands and feet, clenched jaw and grinding teeth, upset stomach including diarrhoea, constipation and nausea.

Cleansing the skin with good hygienic standards in mind. Use pH Balanced skin products to cleanse and moisturise your skin daily. Correct hygiene practices are also very important to preserve good and younger looking skin in life, as discussed in the 'Important Hygienic Practices for Cosmetics And Skin Products' section.

A HEALTHY DIET AND THE DIGESTIVE SYSTEM

A healthy diet promotes overall health in the body that will be reflected on the skin, especially the face. Gut health has a direct influence on the skin. As I have mentioned in the beginning of this book, our face is our image to the world and it tells a story of what is going on in our life. What we eat and how we eat is contributing to our overall health. Outside appearances like our skin, nails, hair, teeth, and eyes will mirror how good our inner health is. I'll explain in the following paragraphs what I mean by this.

We have heard bits and pieces before but, may not get the full picture all at once. Over the years I had a good understanding of healthy eating, but recently did some experimentation and research. All of a sudden I could see the full picture. For some of you the following information that I am going to share is not new, but I am sure for the majority it will make sense for the first time in their life. Without going into too many technical terms, as I am not a qualified doctor, I'll explain it in easy terms as I understand it.

THE HUMAN DIGESTIVE SYSTEM

The main hollow digestive system in our body includes our mouth, oesophagus, stomach, small intestine, large intestine, rectum, and anus. There are organs in our body that also help with digestion such as the pancreas, liver, and gallbladder; but I'll not go into these technical processes. The purpose of this section is to explain correct eating habits and processes for healthy skin and body.

Digestion starts in your *mouth* where you break and chew food into smaller pieces that are more easily digested. Saliva mixes with food to begin the process of breaking it down into a form your body can easily absorb and use. Then the food goes through the throat called the pharynx, moving into the *oesophagus* that is a muscular tube extending from the throat to the stomach. By means of a series of contractions, the oesophagus delivers the food to the stomach. Just before the connection to the stomach, there is a valve preventing the food from passing backwards into the oesophagus.

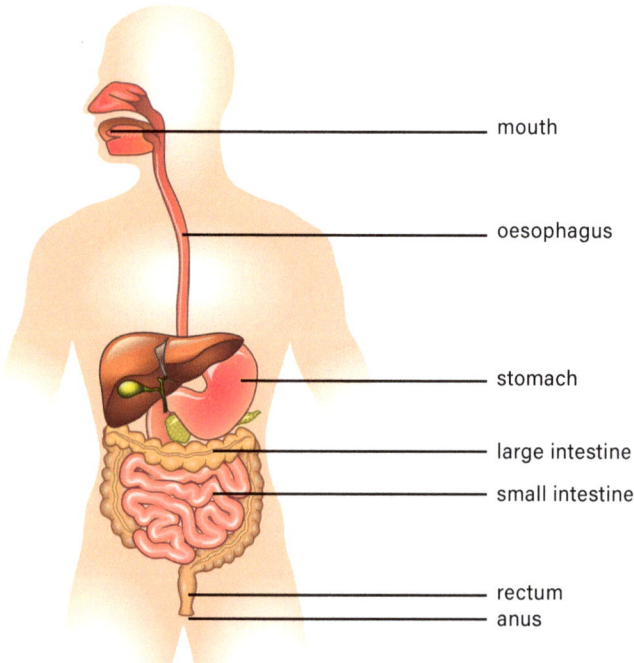

Illustration of the human digestive tract.

The *stomach* is working like a mixer and grinder, secreting acid and powerful enzymes that continue the process of breaking down the food. When the food leaves the stomach, it should be in a consistency of a liquid or paste. From there the food moves to the small intestine.

The *small intestine* is made up of three segments, the duodenum, jejunum, and ileum; continuing the process of breaking down food by using enzymes released by the pancreas and bile from the liver. The first section or duodenum is largely responsible for continuing the process of breaking down food, while the next two sections: jejunum and ileum are mainly responsible for the absorption of nutrients into the bloodstream.

Waste left over from the above digestive processes, is then passing through the *large intestine* or colon by contractions, first in a liquid state and ultimately in solid form as the water is removed from the stool. A stool is stored in the end part of the large intestine until a 'mass movement' empties it into the rectum once or twice a day.

Just a quick and easy explanation, for those who did not know how the digestive system works. The reason why I want you to understand the digestive system is because I have studied it at secondary and tertiary level, and thought I knew it well. But only over the past year a few things made sense on how important is what you eat and how you eat it. A healthy gut will affect our whole body and skin in a positive way. An unhealthy gut will produce illnesses somewhere in the body and reflects negatively on the skin.

The whole journey of me starting to investigate everything was after two years of constant indigestion symptoms, where I got to a point of 'I've had enough'. Medication from the doctor could not cure my symptoms, it only gave me temporarily relief. Even proper surgical procedures such as an endoscopy and gastroscopy could not find anything wrong, or explain why I got heartburn all the time. I am very healthy in general and couldn't figure out why I could not get over these acidity and heartburn feelings in my stomach and oesophagus. It got to a point where I could not even eat or drink nutritional foods that help build a healthy immune system, like apples and oranges. And this was the turning point for me.

Let me say this first, as I have learnt it the hard way, to eat food considered healthy and unhealthy together, is not doing justice to your body. If you eat classified unhealthy food with healthy food, you might as well realise that you are eating unhealthily altogether. The healthy food that you are eating is not going to make the unhealthy food, less unhealthy. Once the unhealthy foods get into your body, it creates a chain of events that causes a lot of different problems or illnesses. We have good and bad bacteria in our body, especially in the digestive tract that gets in contact with the food we eat every day. By not eating enough healthy foods to help build a strong immune system, we become sick quicker, and most likely will cause an overgrowth of bacteria in the body, particular in the digestive tract.

When I was suffering for so long from indigestion, I figured I had nothing to lose and started to treat myself for an overgrowth of bacteria, in particular Helicobacter Pylori and Candida. I am positive there was an overgrowth of other bacteria as well. So I figured if the treatments I am going to follow are going to kill these two bacteria, it will do the others too. Unfortunately by killing bad bacteria, you also kill good bacteria in the process. You'll have to fill it on by taking good bacteria daily in the form of a Probiotic supplement, or foods like: natural yogurt, kefir, kombucha, sauerkraut, dark chocolate, natto, olives, raw cheese, kvass, and miso. I started with a cup of green tea and a teaspoon of active Manuka honey every morning, followed by Mastic Gum tablets that are all known for killing bacteria. Then I waited about two to three hours for it to do its work, before I took my Probiotics with a late breakfast or lunch. There are many different options and before you want to start cleaning yourself from unwanted bacteria, make an appointment at your GP or Naturopath to help you work out the best cleansing routine for you. I'm touching briefly on this for you to understand a few things but will not go in too much detail, as it is a book on its own. And because I have learned from the professionals in their field, I'll refer you to them. I recommend that you also read the following two books: *The H Pylori Diet* by David Hompes and *Dr Gundry's Diet Evolution*.

It took me two months of following the instructions and eating habits in these two books, and I felt like a new person. Could even eat and drink apples and oranges again. I made the decision to make it a lifestyle of eating healthy now and I encourage you to do the same.

What is the problem then with our eating habits today that make us energyless, sick and overweight?

People's busy lives leave them time-poor, and when they are hungry they grab pre-packed foods from the supermarket shelves, or buy fast foods from a café or drive-through. Another factor to blame is that people's taste buds got used to all the comfort foods and when they get hungry they grab these foods first like hamburgers, chips, fizzy drinks, cakes, candy, fried foods, pizza etc. to help get rid of the hunger feeling quickly. The major problem with this kind of diet is that these foods lack proper nutrition the human body so desperately needs for optimum functioning, and the producing of energy.

Eating fast- and pre-packed foods will fill you up and the hungry feeling will temporarily go away. As the food goes through the digestive system, nutrients are absorbed, and the body recognised that the nutritious value is not sufficient. Now the body sends signals that it is hungry again. That is why people keep being hungry.

Modern agricultural methods on the other hand also have stripped increasing amounts of nutrients from the soil and therefore most fruit and vegetables do not have the nutritious value it had in the good old days. Some health enthusiasts produce their own food to make sure it has a higher nutritional value. Fortunately there are some shops, cafes and restaurants that opened over the past few years that are focused on selling and producing good nutritional food. Since research shown how many people get sick of the way they eat, there was a turn on how food needs to be produced and prepared for optimum health benefits. Luckily for us these health enthusiasts stepped out boldly to teach others to make them aware of all the risks factors of eating food with little or no nutritional value.

Most pre-packed and refined foods contain gluten, wheat, salt, sugar, and additives, triggering our taste buds to want more. Videos on social media recently resurfaced showing a chemical used to strip paint from walls as an ingredient in some breakfast cereals. Then you'll also find dodgy ingredients like aluminium in some baking powders, MSG (monosodium glutamate) which is an additive used in food as a flavour enhancer making it more savoury and meaty. Unnatural ingredients in foods build up as toxins in the body proposing huge health risks if constantly eaten. Manufacturers hide obvious dangerous ingredients by only including a number as the ingredient, which will make consumers unaware of the real ingredient. Eating all these unnatural and chemical based ingredients are linked to cancers, tumours, and other illnesses. Do yourself a favour and go through your pantry and research all the ingredients listed on the packaging of foods, and you'll be astonished.

Wheat and gluten is found in all sorts of food like bread, pizzas, pastas, flour, sauces, cereals, cakes, pastries etc. Because it is found in all the foods that most people eat on a daily basis, they do not realise how much they consume every day. Too much of these two ingredients cause undesirable reactions in the human body. For example, wheat has a high glycaemic index causing problems with your blood sugar. The starches within wheat are broken down very quickly and are absorbed into your blood very rapidly, leading to a spike in your blood sugar. This causes a feeling of satisfaction and satiation, but when your blood sugar spikes rapidly, it also drops rapidly. This drop can leave you feeling tired, weak and dizzy. Wheat contains gluten, which is a protein. The consumption of gluten causes symptoms such as bloating, tiredness, headaches and nausea.

Dr. Mark Hyman wrote in an article 'Three hidden ways wheat makes you fat' on his website saying: "The healthy wheat that our ancestors ate is very different from the modern wheat that is available today. Wheat today is a product of genetic manipulation and hybridization that created short, stubby, hardy, high yielding wheat plants with much higher amounts of starch and gluten and many more chromosomes coding for all sorts of new odd proteins. The man who engineered this modern wheat won the Nobel Prize as it promised to feed millions of starving around the world. Well, it has, and it has made them fat and sick."

Sugar again has no nutritional value or benefit to the human body but only a heap of negative reactions that it creates. Read more on sugar's devastating effects that follows.

SUGAR'S DEVASTATING EFFECTS ON THE HUMAN BODY

During my research and experimentations on myself, I realised the following. Our body was designed to eat organic berries, fruits, vegies, and meats. Not the loads of sugary foods and drinks, preservatives, and carbohydrates that convert to sugar during the digestion process. Food supplies have changed dramatically over the past century and we are not eating as we should. That is why we have the obesity epidemic and lots of different diseases that is killing wonderful people.

An article by www.theconversation.com '*The Conversation Academic Rigour, Journalistic Flair in October 2015* showed that the sugarcane is the world's third most valuable crop after cereals and rice, and occupies 26,942,686 hectares of land across the globe. Its main output, apart from commercial profits, is a global public health crisis, which has been centuries in the making.

Human physiology evolved on a diet containing very little sugar and virtually no refined carbohydrates. In fact, sugar probably entered into our diets by accident. It is likely that sugarcane was primarily a 'fodder' crop, used to fatten pigs, though humans may have chewed on the stalks from time to time, to extract its sweetness. Indians discovered how to crystallise sugar during the Gupta dynasty, around 350 AD. The first chemically refined sugar appeared on the scene in India about 2,500 years ago.'

Today about every pre-packed food that we buy contains sugar. Scientists have found that sugar is addictive and stimulates the same pleasure centres of the brain as cocaine or heroin. In short, sugar is just as addictive as cocaine and heroin, and sometimes more. Just like those hard-core drugs, getting off sugar leads to withdrawal and cravings, requiring an actual detox process to wean off. No wonder the world is so hooked on sugar.

Fruit contains fructose, which is metabolised differently than sugar. Therefore it is better to substitute fruits for sugary treats and foods. But again you must have moderation in mind when you ditch sugar and go on to the natural and healthy sugars, such as honey and fruits. Even too much natural sugar can be unhealthy.

Dr. Mark Hyman, creator of the book, *The Blood Sugar Solution 10-Day Detox Diet*, says it only takes 10 days or less to break the addictive cycle of carb and sugar cravings that robs us of our health. When you are done with your 10 days of sugar detox, you'll not crave it so much anymore. Ten days are definitely manageable, don't you think? I have done it, and I challenge you to do it too. It's not that hard but does require a mind change first.

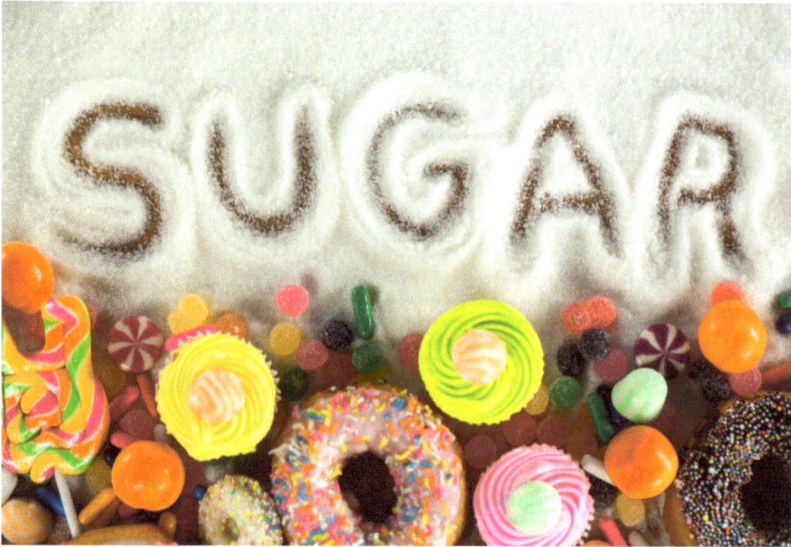

Make today the day to decide enough is enough, and start eating healthier! Only you can make this decision, no one else can make that decision for you successfully. Many people have been put on a diet to lose weight, but afterwards just went back to the weight before their diet, and in some instances they even gained more weight than before. The reason is that they have not made the decision themselves to live a healthier life. Some of you have tried just about every diet there is and could not succeeded, because after the diet you went back to the same old eating habits as before. Complications in the world today are that people consume the following foods on a daily basis: sugar, wheat, gluten, chemically processed foods and meats, genetically modified foods, carbohydrates, soy products, dairy and cheeses.

The more raw fruits and vegies you include in your diet, the better. Another healthy option is to 'quick stir-fry' your vegies so that they still have that crunch. Cut down significantly on potatoes that convert to sugar during the digestion process. The biggest problem of eating sugary foods, potatoes and pastas is, the more you eat them, the more you are going to crave them. Including sugar in your daily diet is not to be taken lightly. It creates havoc in the body. Some negative effects include:

making you hungry that you want to eat more, interfering with your appetite hormones which means your body cannot tell when it is still hungry or full, preventing you from burning fat when you work out at the gym, raises your insulin and as a result programming your body to store more fat. Consuming sugar in large enough amounts can result in a burst of energy known as a 'sugar high', ending in a sharp drop in energy levels called a 'crash'.

Artificial sweeteners again are working more like a pesticide in the body, where they are stored as a toxin because they cannot be broken down. The build-up of toxins in the body cause diseases, kill the friendly bacteria in our gut, block oxygen from binding to red blood cells, block enzymes the body needs for normal functions, block absorption of vitamins and minerals, interfere with DNA synthesis, attack the gut cells, and create holes in the intestinal lining called leaky gut. According to the Pesticide Action Network UK, long term pesticide exposure has been linked to the development of Parkinson's disease, asthma, depression, anxiety, cancer, attention deficit and hyperactivity disorder (ADHD).

Dr. Colbert who created the *Keto Zone Diet* recommends the following natural sweeteners in moderation which are safe: stevia, monk fruit, and sweet alcohols such as erythritol and xylitol.

For the sake of weight loss, you'll have to cut out all sugars and artificial sugars completely from your diet. Use honey and rice malt syrup as alternatives. The simple decision of wanting to live a healthier life, you'll have to change your diet today. Do not delay! The sooner you start, the sooner you'll reap the benefits from it. The amazing truth is that you'll feel and look younger for longer in your life. That is my desire, and I am sure that will be most of you reading this book's desire. Aging gracefully is beautiful and inspiring. Let's inspire our children and grandchildren to age gracefully with us.

Coming back to the bad bacteria that live in our digestion track. They live on sugar, especially the ones in our mouth. By eating sugary food every day and all day long, they'll populate to a stage where they'll become overgrown in the body, and start affecting your overall health in a negative way.

Foods causing inflammation in the body

Apart from injuries or illnesses in our body that causes inflammation, there are more devious culprits in our everyday practices that are silent intruders, robbing the human race from perfect health, and that is some foods that we eat. Research shows that a significant contributor to chronic inflammation comes from what we eat. Chronic inflammation in our body can lead to weight gain, drowsiness, skin problems, digestive issues, all kinds of different diseases, from diabetes to obesity to cancer. Before I started on my healthy living for life, I needed an ice pack on my neck almost every day, just to get rid of the uncomfortable pain and heat. Six months into my healthier eating lifestyle I felt so much better.

The number one inflammatory causing food is no secret by now: sugar. Sugar suppresses the effectiveness of our body's white blood cells that attack and kill germs. Therefore sugar weakens our immune system, making us more susceptible to infectious diseases.

A big number two food that causes inflammation in the body is refined wheat flour, also known as carbohydrates or in short carbs. Refined wheat flour is stripped of its slow-digesting fibre and nutrients, which mean the body can break it down very quickly. Foods falling in this category are pizza bases, white bread, cakes, biscuits, pastas, crackers, breakfast cereals, instant sauces etc. The quicker the body digests these glucose-containing foods, the faster the blood sugar levels spike. This again causes insulin levels to spike, which is a compound associated with a pro-inflammatory response.

Thirdly are dairy products such as milk, cheese, yogurt, and butter. Dairy is a common allergen that triggers inflammatory reactions through the release of histamines in the body. One in four adults have difficulty digesting milk, whether they are lactose intolerant, or have sensitivity to its casein proteins. If you feel particularly bloated after consuming dairy, you might consider cutting dairy from your diet. Calcium can be included in your diet through other foods like broccoli, spinach, kale, rhubarb, beans and lentils, sunflower seeds, green beans, baby carrots, sardines, sesame seeds, almonds, oranges, sweet potatoes, green leave vegetables, fresh blackberries, dried apricots, and dried figs.

Fourth, are artificial sweeteners that disrupt the composition of our gut microbiota by decreasing levels of the good bacteria Bacteroides, which are known to help release anti-inflammatory compounds. All foods, candy and drinks claiming there is no sugar in, most likely contain artificial sweeteners.

Fifth, are artificial additives that enhance the taste, smell and colour of a food. Common culprits are breakfast cereals, ice creams, candy, processed foods containing fruits. Artificial also means not found naturally in nature. Artificial colouring is made from petroleum that has been implicated as a host for different health issues, from disrupting hormone function that causes hyperactivity in children to tumour production in animal studies.

Sixth, are saturated fats found in hamburgers, chips, pizzas, and candy. Multiple studies have connected saturated fats with the triggering of white adipose tissue or fat tissue inflammation. This white tissue is the type of fat that stores energy, rather than burns energy like brown fat cells do. According to a review in the journal Expert Review of Cardiovascular Therapy, when your fat cells get bigger with greater intakes of saturated fats, they release pro-inflammatory agents that promote systemic inflammation.

Seventh, are fried foods such as French fries, fried chicken tenders and fish sticks, and fried onion rings. Vegetable-oil-fried and processed foods contain high levels of inflammatory advanced glycation end products (AGEs), when they are cooked at high temperatures, pasteurised, dried, smoked, fried, or grilled. Researchers from the Mount Sinai School of Medicine found that when people cut out processed and fried foods that have high levels of AGEs, markers of inflammation in their body diminished.

Eighth are grain-fed meats like beef, lamb, pork, and chicken. Because the animals did not evolve on a grain-fed diet, many producers have to load up the animals with antibiotics. These drugs keep the animals from getting diseases in cramped feedlots or getting sick from their unnatural diet, and also help them gain weight faster, which again have a direct link to humans eating these meats, gaining weight faster as well. Altogether, this means people who are eating these meats that are higher in inflammatory saturated fats, have greater levels of inflammatory omega-6s from the corn and soy diet. The human body is then in a constant state of attack, due to ingesting leftover levels of antibiotics and hormones.

Coming to number nine are processed meats that include cold meats, bacon, bologna, sausages, and jerky. They are made from meats that are high in saturated fats, containing high levels of advanced glycation end products (AGEs). These inflammatory compounds are created when these processed meats are dried, smoked, pasteurised, and cooked at high temperatures. A lot of times they are also injected with lots of preservatives, colourings, and artificial flavourings that attack our immune system.

Number ten is the ingredient gluten found in bread, pizza bases, pastas, crackers, seasonings and mixed spices are made from refined white flour. Many of the breads on the market go from flour and yeast to baked bread in just a few hours. This shortening period of fermentation causes a decrease in the amount of starch and gluten the yeast typically can pre-digest for us. Without the assistance in digestion, it can be harder for our bodies to digest the bread's gluten, causing inflammation in the lining of our intestines.

Number eleven is alcohol including wine, beers, and liquors. The process of breaking down alcohol generates toxic by-products that can damage liver cells, promote inflammation, and weaken the body's immune system. According to a study published in the journal Toxicology, the flavonoids and antioxidants found in red wines and the probiotics in beer, might actually contribute an anti-inflammatory effect. But as we all know, too much alcohol has a string of negative effects on the body. Hard liquors are even more harmful and toxic for your body than the so called low alcohol content drinks.

Number twelve is using all kinds of medication to help you feel better. For example; painkillers for a headache; medications to relieve acid reflux, ulcers, and heartburn; medication for nausea, skin rushes etc. Rather than popping a pill to get rid of your ailments, try a natural remedy first. Read a few of my natural remedies for pains and aches a bit further on.

Feeling and being healthy therefore is all in your reach, if you are mindful of what you pop into your mouth. Some people have said to me it is hard to make the transition. And yes, I agree it is hard to get to that point where you say no more of bad eating. The secret of succeeding is, renewing of your mind and giving yourself at least a month to wean your body off all these slowly killing ingredients. For most people a sudden change in their diet fails because the toxic and addictive ingredients are still in the body, and when they suddenly stop eating them, the cravings get worse.

For a smooth transition from eating very unhealthy to healthy, start cutting out more of these addictive foods every day. For example, if you are used to drinking three teaspoons of sugar in your coffee or tea, cut down immediately to two teaspoons of sugars for a week. Then cut down to one teaspoon of sugar the following week, followed by no sugar the week after. Alternatively change over to a teaspoon of honey straight away in your tea or coffee, and also cut down on the amounts of cups you drink during the day. Do the same with all the other unhealthy foods and drinks, so that after a month you can cut it out altogether and start to eat only healthy ingredients. This way it will not be such a shock to your body. You can also go on a detox diet straight away to get rid of these toxic ingredients in the body sooner, which will bring you closer to feeling better. I recommend that you make an appointment with your general practitioner, naturopath, or qualified dietician, to help you through this process of detoxification. This way it is done correctly with minimal risks to whatever your body may experience. Always check with your general practitioner first before you make drastic changes to your diet.

THE CORRECT WAY TO EAT YOUR FOOD FOR OPTIMAL HEALTH

For optimum health it is important how we eat our food too. Where possible eat your fruit and vegies raw, but make sure you wash them properly to ensure that they are clean from pesticides and bacteria on the outside. Peeling or cooking also removes bacteria. Do not wash fresh produce with soaps or detergents though because if you did not rinse off all the soap, you run the risk of eating the soap again that becomes another toxin for the body. For one to two fruits, just simply wash it under a running tap of clean drinkable water. More fruits can be placed in a bowl with cold clean drinkable water, then wash each fruit or vegie separately, before placing it in a clean plate or bowl. Use a vegetable brush, to brush away hard-to-remove microbes from produce with thick skin. Veggies with a lot of nooks and crannies like cauliflower, broccoli or lettuce should be soaked for two to five minutes in a bowl with clean water, and a half teaspoon of table salt added to the water.

The next important practice is to chew your food as many times as possible, before swallowing it. The physical process of chewing food in your mouth helps to break down larger particles of food into smaller particles. This helps to reduce stress on the oesophagus and the stomach. Chewing each mouthful properly, will release enough saliva that contains digestive enzymes. When your food isn't digested properly, you could suffer from digestive issues such as indigestion, heartburn, constipation, headaches and low energy.

Proper chewing will also reduce the risk of bacterial overgrowth in the digestive tract, especially in the colon, that will lead to nasty indigestion issues. Releasing enough saliva relaxes the lower stomach and speeds up the digestive process. According to the experts at Ohio State University, you should chew softer foods five to ten times, and more dense foods like meats and vegetables up to 30 times before swallowing. Beverages with a meal would never be used if people took the time to thoroughly chew their food. Washing food down and diluting the digestive juices with fluids, always result in only partial digestion of the food.

If weight loss is your goal, a Chinese study published in the *American Journal of Clinical Nutrition* reported that a person needs to chew food at least 40 times per bite before swallowing. Most experts say to simply chew your food until it has lost all its texture or liquefied in your mouth. Chewing correctly helps your body from the start to extract the most nutrition from the food, and the best nutrition will continue to be released right through the digestive process. One great benefit is that it will take the extra workload off your stomach and intestines, so they do not have to work harder to digest the food.

To improve digestion and reducing the risk of constipation and bloating, avoid drinking water or beverages while eating. Too much liquid in the stomach dilute the digestive fluids and slow down digestion. However, you can drink up to 20-30 minutes before or after your meal, to avoid dehydration.

Be conscious of what you pop in your mouth every minute of every day. This will not just ensure that you are healthier and staying in shape, but promote clear, glowing skin. Some signs for you to know that your diet is not producing the nutrients your body needs to operate sufficiently are, when you stay hungry during the day and you crave quick energy boosters such as chocolates, hamburgers, fried chips, sweets, fizzy drinks etc. By eating a healthy diet every day, and chewing it the right way, you'll notice that you will feel fuller for longer. You'll look at the clock and think 'Oh it is time to eat', because you usually eat something at that time of the day. But your body will signal 'I am not hungry; please do not feed me now'.

Drink warm to room temperature beverages, as too cold and too hot drinks are harmful for the body. An ice cold drink with a meal can completely halt the digestive process. The inside of the body is a delicate, well-controlled environment, where digestion proceeds at a proper pace when this environment is kept constant. Pouring a glass of ice cold water into the stomach while eating, is like taking food that is cooking in the oven and sticking it into a freezer, suspending the cooking process. That is how the digestive process is suspended when drinking cold beverages while eating. Nerve endings are numbed by intense cold just as they are numbed by very hot beverages. Drinking cold water shrinks blood vessels, weakening your immune system, and causes indigestion.

Hot drinks that are above 104 degrees will destroy the sensitive nerve endings in the tongue. They benumb the senses so that discrimination of taste is lost. They scar the oesophagus and stomach lining, disrupt body temperature and digestion. Drink warm or room temperature water to keep health issues at bay.

What about salt? What we know as salt is really sodium chloride. It is forty per cent sodium and the rest is chlorine. Sea salt, rock salt and table salt all contain around one hundred per cent sodium chloride, which means that too much of any of them will have a negative effect on your health. Table salt is rock salt that has been finely grounded and can be iodized, or have iodine added to it, but the sodium chloride content of both is the same. Iodine is a critical micronutrient in the human diet because our bodies cannot synthesize that, so we have to rely on food to obtain it. The iodine in iodized salt helps the body make a thyroid hormone that is critical to an infant's brain development.

Rock salt and sea salt are often marketed as being a healthier or tastier option than table salt, and can be considerably more expensive than table salt. Sea salt is produced by the evaporation of sea water. It is argued that sea salt contains more minerals than table salt so is better for your health. Just because it may contain extra minerals does not mean it is good for you.

Everyone needs salt for fluid balance, muscle and nerve functioning. Too little sodium can lead to hyponatremia, and symptoms of dizziness, confusion, muscle twitches and seizures. Too much sodium has been linked to kidney stones, high blood pressure, and cardiovascular disease. In general, small amounts of salt are essential to our health. Adults need less than one gram per day and children need even less. If your doctor said you have to stay away from salt due to an illness, you'll have to comply. A high salt diet can raise your blood pressure, leading to heart attacks and strokes.

Probably the most important determinant factor of your health is what you eat. The food you eat every day makes up how you look, how you feel, how much energy you have, and how you spend the rest of your life. That is why being food conscious is really necessary for optimum health. Stay away from junk food, preservatives, pesticides, sugar and sugary foods, pickled food, canned food, wheat and gluten. Eat organic and fresh as much as possible, and you will feel the remarkable difference.

EATING THE WRONG COMBINATIONS OF FOODS

Something else I have discovered is that there are certain foods that you should not eat together. Some food combinations can affect our body badly. They can overload the stomach, resulting in inhibition of enzyme systems, and the production of toxins. When the same foods are eaten separately, they are not only digested quicker, but also provide more energy for the body. An obvious example is that meats will take longer to digest than fruits. Fruits contain simple sugars that require almost no digestion and when eaten with meat, the fruit sugar will stay too long in the stomach and ferment, resulting in gas and bloating.

A basic rule is to eat fruit on an empty stomach, to allow efficient digestion. Do not combine protein (meat, poultry, eggs, cheese and fish) and starches (oats, rice, pasta, bread, potato, corn etc.) in the same meal either. The simple explanation is, there are different enzymes in the body that help digest protein and carbohydrates, if you eat them together it will cause digestive issues. Eating foods together that have different digestion speeds will leave you with partially digested food in your digestive system that just sits there in your gut, while the other foods are being digested. During this waiting period the partially digested food will rot or ferment, causing bloating, gas, constipation or diarrhoea.

In all my years I have never known that there are foods that should not be eaten together. In the process of starting to be healthier, I felt so much better. But I realised again there were days that I did not feel as healthy as I ate. A thought came up in my mind 'maybe there are foods that cannot be eaten together'. That is where my research started again. Founding out that indeed some foods should not be eaten together. While the medical and nutrition fields are divided on the food combining principles, I think people need to judge for themselves. When a person is not feeling that well they will try just anything to feel healthy and better again. That is what I did! I have experimented with food combining to see how my body feels afterwards.

We are all falling in different age groups and have different body sizes, we have distinctive blood types, and have our favourite foods that we eat on a regular basis, giving us a certain pH on the inside of our body. As we are getting older, the pH level of our body also changes, and when we get to a certain age we realise that some foods that we used to eat when we were younger, now affect our well-being. I believe that one rule does not fit all. Each person needs to judge how they are feeling after they have eaten a certain food or meal. The amount of advice out there is plenty from professionals and health enthusiasts. But the only person who can really tell you how you feel is yourself.

From my childhood I just loved acidic and sour foods and could not get enough of it. For example, I only drank Rooibos tea with freshly squeezed lemon juice, tomatoes were in almost every meal, sour apples and pine apples were my favourite, and of course I had an orange or apple juice about every day. Reaching my late forties, I realised I cannot eat like that anymore and had to adjust my diet. At the end of the day the best way for you is, to test and trial what is working for you.

I have trialed food combining on myself, and I am feeling so much healthier. Evidence suggests that attention to food combining may not be necessary for people with good digestion. When you eat well and still struggle with indigestion, gas, bloating, heartburn; you are better off to book an appointment at a professional, to get to the bottom of your symptoms. To be hundred percent safe is to do this under the supervision of a professional, especially when you are working through an illness. Always consult your general practitioner or nutritionist before changing your diet significantly. Following are some undesirable reactions caused in the body by combining the wrong foods:

- *Indigestion*: pain or discomfort in the stomach associated with difficulty in digesting food.

- *Producing of toxins*: a toxin is anything that damages the body. Toxins can be from food (gluten, wheat, legumes, etc.), the air, water, mould, clothing, or for some, even their cell phone. Buy food that is free from preservatives, chemicals, and colouring agents. Choose chemical-free and organic varieties where possible.

- *Fermentation*: the chemical breakdown of a substance by bacteria, yeasts, or other microorganisms, typically involving effervescence and the giving off of heat.

- *Gas and bloating*: the abdomen feels full, tight, or swollen. Abdominal bloating occurs when the digestive tract is filled with air or gas.

- *Putrefaction*: the process of decay or rotting in a body or other organic matter.

- *Eating the wrong foods for prolonged periods can lead to toxaemia and disease*: toxaemia is blood poisoning by toxins from a local bacterial infection. Long term diseases can be bad breath, dry skin, rashes, chronic inflammation, poor sleep, low energy, and chronic digestion issues.

FOODS RECOMMENDED NOT TO COMBINE IN ONE MEAL

- *Eat fruits alone and on an empty stomach*: Separate acidic and sweet fruits and do not eat them together. Bananas are a staple of most smoothie recipes. They are sweet and should not be combined with citrus, pineapple, pomegranate or any other sour fruit. Never eat fruit straight after a meal, especially after proteins and starches. Fruit does not require major digestion due to the natural sugar it contains. Eating them together will cause gas, bloating, and the potential for developing an upset stomach. Do not eat watermelon with anything else either, because it doesn't digest well with any other food, including other fruits. When you have a weak stomach, avoid eating very acidic fruits on an empty stomach.

- *Do not eat protein and starches together*: Digesting protein and starch requires different enzymes and other chemicals. To digest each most effectively, they need to be eaten separately. Proteins include: red meat, chicken, fish, seafood, eggs, nuts, seeds, tofu, legumes such as beans, peas and lentils. Starches include: grains, potatoes, breads, pasta, rice, wheat, maize, flour, corn.

- *Bananas and milk*: Various experts have stated that this combination is very heavy and some people argue that it produces some form of toxin, although this is still disputed. The problem is that this combination is very difficult to digest as it will sit in the stomach for some considerable period of time. If you want to have a smoothie with this combination, make sure that the banana is as ripe as possible.

- *Yogurt and sour fruits*: There are a number of reasons as to why you should not have this as a treat. It is mainly sour fruits that are the issue here. The theory is that it can change the intestinal flora that can lead to all kinds of stomach issues. You can avoid this problem by eating unflavoured yogurt at room temperature and mix in honey, raisins or cinnamon instead of fresh fruit.

- *Water with any meal*: Water might help the food to go down your throat, but the problem is that it goes straight through the system, and in the process dilutes the digestive juices and enzymes that your body requires to digest the food. This means that your body is going to find it harder to digest your meal, and once again, sit there for an extended period of time. Leading to a build-up of gas and making you feel uncomfortable.

- *Cereal or oatmeal with milk and orange juice*: The acids in orange juice or any acid fruits, destroy the enzyme that is responsible for digesting starches present in cereal. They can curdle milk and turn it into a heavy mucus-forming substance. To keep your breakfast healthy, have fruit or orange juice 30 minutes before eating oatmeal.

- *Lemon dressing, cucumber and tomato salad*: Nightshade fruits and vegetables such as tomatoes, potatoes, chillies, and eggplant are not supposed to be combined with cucumbers.

(The term 'nightshade' may have been coined because some of these plants prefer to grow in shady areas, and some flower at night.). While lemon dressing does not go well with cucumber and tomatoes.

- *Beans and cheese*: Beans and dairy protein are a common combination in Mexican dishes. Eaten with a hearty serving of guacamole and hot sauce, they almost guaranteed to lead to gas and bloating. It is not the beans on their own that cause it, but the combination of these two foods. Try skipping cheese and tomatoes if you have a weak digestion.

- *Cheese and meat omelette*: Protein combinations are not recommended. One single concentrated protein per meal is easier to digest and won't require as much energy. Go for a veggie omelette instead.

- *Bacon and eggs*: Two high protein sources take a long time to digest. It is recommended to eat your meals in courses. Eat the light proteins first, followed by the heavier meat later. Never wait longer than 10 minutes between each course.

- *Tomato and cheese*: Tomatoes and cheese are popular foods that people love to combine in meals. Think pastas, pizzas, sandwiches, and salads. Combining an acidic food like tomato, with pasta that is a carbohydrate, is one of the worst food combinations ever. Then adding cheese to it is a recipe for disaster. If you are feeling tired after a meal of tomato, cheese and pasta, don't be surprised. It is because your body requires a lot of energy to digest it.

- *Animal protein with a starch*: This is not the best food combination for your stomach either. Traditional meat and potatoes together are actually bad for your digestion because of how the different digestive juices are created, which counteract one another during the digestion process. The main problem here is that it is going to lead them fermenting in the stomach and ultimately leads to a lot of gas in your intestines.

Dr. Kaslow writes on his website that "a combination of high protein and high starches inhibit the absorption of all the nutritive factors of foods and results in an unnecessary burden upon the entire digestive apparatus. It is well known that many illnesses are due to deficiencies of certain essential food factors such as vitamins and minerals. These deficiencies produce degeneration of certain tissues, and this degeneration results in loss of resistance. Infections then invade us and produce disease. It is not enough to have the essential elements in the food we eat, they must actually be utilised by our bodies, and be available to our tissues. Thus, it is possible to eat large quantities of nutritious foods and get no benefit at all from them, if we eat other foods at the same time that interfere with the proper digestion of vitamin and mineral bearing foods.

When we eat cheese that is rich in calcium, by the time it reaches our small intestine, an alkaline digestive process is going on there, then very little (if any) of that calcium will be available to us. The calcium will make a chemical combination with the alkali and become non-absorbable; it will pass through and out of our body unused! No matter how much cheese we eat, we may still suffer from calcium deficiency, if the calcium does not get absorbed. But if this food reaches the small intestine when an acid condition is present, much of the calcium will be utilised. Obviously then, we must be certain that when we eat cheese, our small intestine will be acid and not alkaline. But how? The answer is clear and incontrovertible. By not eating any high carbohydrates at the same time.

When we eat carbohydrates like starches and sugars, our small intestine becomes alkaline, and a condition is created by which essential factors in other foods cannot be used. These same carbohydrates may interfere with the digestion of certain proteins in the stomach itself, and partially digested protein food will then become toxic material."

If you suffer from a heart disease, I suggest that you read *Dr. Colbert's Keto Zone Diet* book, where he explains why you must not cut out all natural fats from your diet. In fact, natural fats are necessary to repair and improve certain heart conditions. The worst offender in a diet for a heart patient is actually carbohydrates that include sugar and starches. The keto zone diet is not a traditional diet where you follow it for a short while, and then slip back into your old eating habits after it. This diet is a lifestyle eating pattern with lifelong health benefits. Illnesses on this diet either disappear or improve dramatically. Even some of Dr. Colbert's cancer patients have been healed from going on the keto zone lifestyle diet. He also says that by including more healthy fats in your diet, and much-less to-no-carbohydrates, this will make you feel fuller for longer during the day, while you are losing weight. Healthy fats help burn belly fat. The caloric intake of the Keto Zone Diet consists of seventy per cent healthy fats, fifteen per cent green veggies, and fifteen per cent healthy protein. In his book he also gives delicious healthy food recipes. By eating more healthy fats, your skin will look amazing and you will definitely look younger for longer. Foods classified as healthy fats are: extra virgin olive oil, grass-fed butter, coconut and coconut oil, fish oil, avocado oil, avocado, whole egg, fatty fish, dark chocolate, nuts (like almonds, pecans, and macadamia. Raw are better).

I know what you may be thinking now: how can someone recommend what these doctors and professionals are suggesting we eat, if they are not practicing what they are preaching? My answer is 'Yes, I am eating what these doctors suggest and I can promise you it is working'.

FRESH JUICES AND HEALTHY TONIC RECIPES FOR HEALTHY BODY AND SKIN

The following two juices and tonic are what I drink regularly. I would not suggest you drink it every day for the rest of your life, because too much of a good thing can also cause a negative reaction. When I make the *immunity booster* for instance, I drink a glass per day for the following two days while it is still fresh. I'll make this *immunity booster* every seventh day, to have my weekly dose of Vitamin C. When oranges are out of season, I'll just juice carrots diluted with filtered water.

I'll make the *overall health booster tonic* from ginger and cinnamon, and drink a small glass per day for consecutive five to seven days. Then two to four weeks will pass before I make my next batch of the *overall health booster tonic*. And the *energy booster* which is made from watermelon and berries is a drink that I make when these fruits are in season. I'll make myself a fresh glass of this every day in a George Foreman mix-and-go blender. Buying a whole watermelon in season is cheaper. I will cut it in half and cover one half with cling wrap before placing it back in the fridge. When you are keeping the watermelon in its skin, it stays fresher and crunchier for longer. I'll then chop the other half of the watermelon up into big pieces, and store it in a container that has a strainer at the bottom, so that the watermelon does not lie in its own juice. These few easy tips prevent the watermelon from going off quickly.

Immunity Booster

Ingredients

3 x large carrots

2 x juicy oranges

250 ml filtered
drinking water

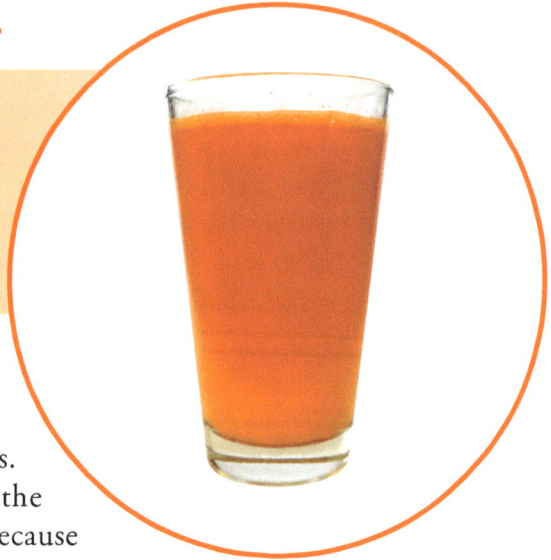

Method:

Juice the carrots and oranges.
Mix together and dilute the
juice with filtered water. Because
of the high fibre content, this can cause
stomach upset and discomfort. The heathiest way to drink this is at
room temperature. To avoid any bloating and discomfort, drink the
immunity booster slowly and in small amounts, only 250 ml at a time.
Don't drink it late at night to avoid feeling bloated and uncomfortable
when going to bed.

TIP: TO PREVENT YOUR TEETH FROM BEING STAINED, DRINK
THIS JUICE WITH A STRAW.

Carrots and oranges are loaded with Vitamin C that helps boost your
body's immunity system, protecting the cells by neutralising free radicals.
Free radicals cause chronic diseases, like cancer and heart disease. It also
protects against viral infections and certain cancers. Beta-carotene in
carrots protects the skin from free radicals and helps prevent the signs
of aging. Vitamin C aids in good eye health and protects vision. They
are also a very good source of dietary fibre, preventing constipation, and
lowering the risk of other diseases.

Energy Booster

Ingredients

¼ of a small seedless watermelon

½ cup of mix berries (blue berries, mulberries and/or raspberries)

½ cup of filtered water

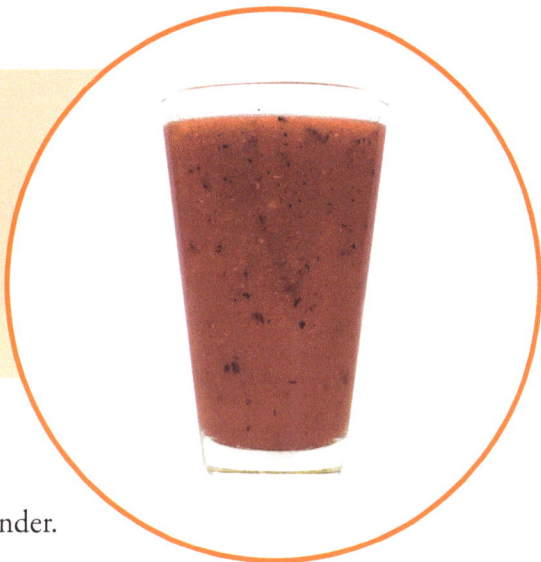

Method:

Put everything through a blender.

TIP: TO PREVENT YOUR TEETH FROM STAINING, DRINK THIS JUICE WITH A STRAW.

A watermelon consists of ninety two per cent water, and contains a lot of nutrients. Watermelon has more lycopene than raw tomatoes. Lycopene is a powerful carotenoid antioxidant that gives fruits and vegetables a pink or red colour. Lycopene is most often associated with tomatoes, but watermelon is actually a more concentrated source of it. Watermelons are rich in anti-inflammatory substances and may significantly reduce blood pressure. Watermelons are also a rich source of Vitamin C that helps your immune system produce antibodies to fight diseases. Berries are amongst the healthiest foods you can eat according to researchers and nutritionists. They contain antioxidants that help keep free radicals under control, fighting inflammation. Berries are good for your skin. In addition to lowering cholesterol, berries provide other benefits for heart health. One of these is better functioning of your arteries.

113

Overall Health Booster Tonic

Ingredients

1 x cinnamon stick

1 x small piece of ginger (2cm² piece)

1lt of filtered water

Small teapot with a little inside drainer

2 x 500 ml glass bottles with a tight lid

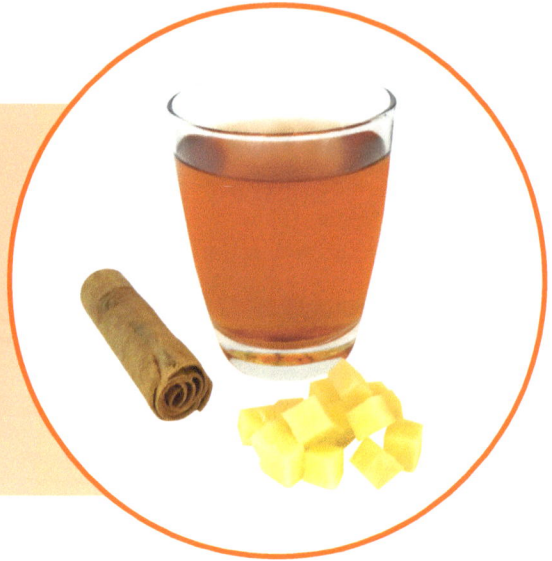

Method:

1. Bring 500 ml of filtered water and the cinnamon stick to boil in a pot. When boiling, turn the heat down and simmer for five-ten minutes. Remove from the stove and place it on a marble or wooden board to cool down. When cooled, pour through a fine sift to remove any small wooden pieces of the cinnamon stick.

2. Boil the other 500 ml of water while peeling the ginger and cut it up in small cubes. Put the ginger cubes inside the drainer of the teapot. Now pour the 500 ml boiled water over the ginger. Let it stand to cool down.

3. When cooled down fill, each 500 ml glass bottle, one with the cinnamon water and the other one with the ginger water.

4. Mix the two tonics to fill up half of a small glass (about 80-100 ml) to drink every day. It is recommended that you drink this early in the morning on an empty stomach.

Ginger has a very long history of use in various forms of traditional or alternative medicine. It has been used to help digestion, reduce nausea and morning sickness, it helps fight the flu and common cold, and reduce muscle pain and soreness. It has an anti-inflammatory effect and may drastically lower blood sugars, improve heart disease risk factors, and can help treat chronic indigestion. Cinnamon is one of the most delicious and healthiest spices on the planet with powerful medicinal properties. It is loaded with antioxidants, has anti-inflammatory properties, and may cut the risk of heart disease, lowers blood sugar levels, may protect against cancer, fight bacterial and fungal infections.

ELLEN'S HEALTHY FOOD OPTIONS AND RECIPES

Who says eating healthily is boring? I'll be honest with you. There is nothing boring about eating healthily. You only have to get used to the new tastes. The longer we eat healthier foods, the better they taste. Researchers have found that it takes one month to train your taste buds to enjoy new tastes, when you cut out the old unhealthy foods. Our taste buds are replaced with new ones every ten to fourteen days.

The other important fact to note is that when you add enough protein and natural fats to your diet, you will feel fuller for longer. You'll not crave quick unhealthy energy boosters such as sugars, carbohydrates, and fast foods so much anymore. Over the years breakfast cereal companies have conditioned our minds to think that a breakfast cereal is the way to start your day. But they are full of unhealthy sugars. Sugar give you a quick boost of energy, then causing blood sugar levels to drop, robbing you of the energy that your deserve to enable you to have an energetic day.

When I started my healthy diet I found that when I started with a healthy protein-based breakfast, I stayed fuller for longer, just as the doctors and experts whose advice I followed promised. Most days, I'll only eat two proper meals per day. But be careful not to eat two proteins together though, because as I have explained in the 'Foods recommended to not combine in one meal', they have different digesting times and can cause bloating when eaten together. You can eat a light protein like fish first, followed by a heavier meat like sausage or steak later. Never wait longer than 10-15 minutes between each course. The popular bacon, eggs, and sausages combination for breakfast will also not help your waistline if you are trying hard to lose the extra kilos.

We all have our own style of eating that we have grown used to over the years. I found that was why it was hard for me to get used to another person's healthy recipes. Then I thought: 'What if I only replace unhealthy ingredients with healthy ingredients in my own recipes that I love?'. And that is what I did, and it became easier for me to stay on the healthy diet. If you find it hard to get used to all the healthy recipes out there as well, start experimenting with your own recipes and make them healthier. We all have our own favourite recipes. For example, my favourite sponge chocolate cake is a recipe that I loved and everybody who had a piece always complimented me on its taste, and asked for the recipe. I have replaced the normal self-raising cake flour in this recipe with gluten and wheat free flour. I bought a healthier baking powder that does not include aluminium as an ingredient. The sunflower oil in the recipe was replaced with coconut oil or olive oil. Sugar in the recipe was replaced with coconut sugar, rice malt syrup and/or honey. I also bought the healthier cacao and vanilla essence versions that includes organic ingredients. Then I add organic eggs. Even the icing for the cake has no sugar in it. My new chocolate sponge cake tastes really good, not as sweet as before, but still sweet enough. This is because I have trained my taste buds to be satisfied with more subtle sweet tastes.

Another factor that can be discouraging when you embark on your new diet and life is that you must start all over in the planning of your weekly grocery shopping. You have to learn how much to buy, and where to find all these new healthy ingredients. Food shopping for the first few months will take much longer because you need to figure out which shelves to find the healthy products on. Hang in there! You'll get to the point again when food shopping and food recipes are easy. And I promise you that it will all be worth it in the end when you feel and look healthier. You'll also find that when you eat healthy foods, your body will extract more nutrients from the food, and you'll not require that much food every day.

To save time and food, I'll wash half of a lettuce and store it in a salad bowl that has a drainer at the bottom, so that the lettuce does not lie in the water at the bottom of the bowl. When lettuce lies in water for a few days it goes off quicker. When you grate half of a carrot, store the other half of the carrot in the same bowl as the lettuce. So when you need to make your next salad, it happens quickly because the ingredients are already washed and prepared. Every time you use half of an avocado, store the other half in a small container with a few drops of lemon on the flesh to prevent it from oxidising quickly.

The following are a few of my food combinations and recipes that work well.

BREAKFAST OPTIONS

1. Natural and healthy wrap sheet with natural healthy ingredients: mashed avocado, lettuce, a handful of baby spinach, grated carrot,

sliced cucumber, three fish fingers or chicken tenders (try the ones with a gluten free coating).

2. Cooked salmon, half of an avocado, handful of baby spinach, handful of walnuts, beetroot.

3. Four slices of corn Cruskits, one avocado, mashed, two boiled eggs, sliced. Spread the smashed avocado on each Cruskit and place the sliced eggs on top. Season to taste.

4. A salad with the following ingredients: Lettuce, baby spinach, half of an avocado sliced, eight thin slices of cucumber, two boiled eggs cut in quarter wedges (boiled eggs can also be replaced with fish or chicken).

5. Omelette, made with two eggs and the following filling: fried onions and two mushrooms, one small banana cut in wheels. See my recipe further on. This is a beautiful taste together, but because you are eating a fruit and protein together, ensure you are chewing each bite well so that the digestion in the mouth starts well.

6. Bowl of organic cooked oats, teaspoon of grass-fed butter, 1 teaspoon of honey, small banana cut into wheels, almond milk.

7. Healthy ingredients pancakes, with rice malt syrup. See my recipe further down.

8. Slice of healthy carrot cake made with healthy ingredients. (Gluten and wheat free flour, no sugar but rice malt syrup and/or honey).

9. Sushi without any soy sauce. Add salt and lemon for extra taste. It is healthier to make your own sushi. Sushi can be left overnight in the fridge and will still be fresh the next day.

10. Maize meal or polenta porridge with beef sausage. See my maize meal recipe further on.

11. Bowl of organic natural yoghurt or coconut yoghurt with honey and walnuts.

12. Bowl of organic natural yoghurt or coconut yoghurt with muesli.

13. Watermelon and blue berries.

Lunch and Dinner Options

1. Salmon with stir-fried veggies like carrots, string beans, mushrooms, onion, cauliflower, and broccoli. You can also add a fresh garden salad on the side.

2. Freshly made meatballs or any of your favourite meat like chops, T-bone, or chicken, with stir-fry veggies, and a garden salad.

3. Pan-fried chops, gluten and wheat free gravy sauce, roasted pumpkin and boiled peas.

4. Gluten and wheat free pizza with all healthy toppings excluding salami and processed meats.

5. Gluten and wheat free spaghetti with a topping of fried lean mince-meat, mushrooms, onion, and garlic. Add gluten and wheat free gravy sauce or freshly made tomato sauce if you love your sauce. Serve it with beetroot and a garden salad.

6. Marinate 10-12 pieces of chicken sirloins for a couple of hours in half of an orange freshly squeezed, 2-4 tablespoons of honey. Pan fries the sirloin till it is golden brown and eat it with a green salad including string beans, baby spinach, lettuce, avocado.

7. If you are craving French fries rather make the following alternative every once in a while: Peel two red skinned potatoes and cut it in small cubes, then fry in a stick free pan or pot with a little bit of olive oil on a medium heat, turning the potato cubes every 3-4 minutes until golden brown. Enjoy with salt and vinegar/lemon.

8. Meat and veggie soup. In a large pot, fry 250-500 grams of meat in a bit of olive oil over medium heat and add the onion and garlic clove a bit later (the meat can be mince, lamb cubes, gravy meat, or lamb cutlets). While the meat is cooking in the pot for about 20-30 minutes on low to medium heat, prepare the veggies. Cut the broccoli pieces from the main stem and soak in salt water, peel two large carrots and two large red skinned potatoes and grate them together, then add to the meat in the pot with half a kettle of boiling water, close the lid. Wash a bunch of string beans and cut up into small pieces, also cut up the broccoli into smaller pieces. Now add

the broccoli and string beans to the soup pot and add more boiling water so that the veggies have enough room to cook slowly. Add salt and pepper to taste and cook for a further hour. Let the soup cool down for about 15-30 minutes before serving. You can mash the veggies if you prefer a more liquidly soup.

9. Homemade hamburger patties topped with fried tomato, mushrooms, and onion. Serve it with a Greek salad.

10. Lasagne made with gluten and wheat free pasta sheets, served with beetroot and a garden salad.

SNACKS FOR IN BETWEEN MEALS OR ONE HOUR AFTER A MEAL:

1. Any fresh fruit.

2. Half a cup of mixed nuts and dried fruits.

3. Homemade mango ice cream (put two large ripe mangoes in a blender and add two-four tablespoons of coconut milk). Freeze in the freezer. Defrost 15-30 minutes before serving with my pancake recipe or chocolate sponge cake recipe.

4. Small cup of organic natural or coconut yoghurt with honey and walnuts or muesli.

5. A ripe mango cut into cubes served with organic natural or coconut yoghurt.

6. Small piece of organic dark chocolate with 70 per cent plus cacao.

7. Veggie chips.

8. Gluten and wheat free ginger biscuits made with organic ingredients and honey or rice malt syrup.

9. Fresh fruit smoothie.

10. Green tea, rooibos tea, white strawberry tea, or any other organic tea.

Following are a few of my favourite recipes that I make regularly.

ELLEN'S RECIPES

Pancakes

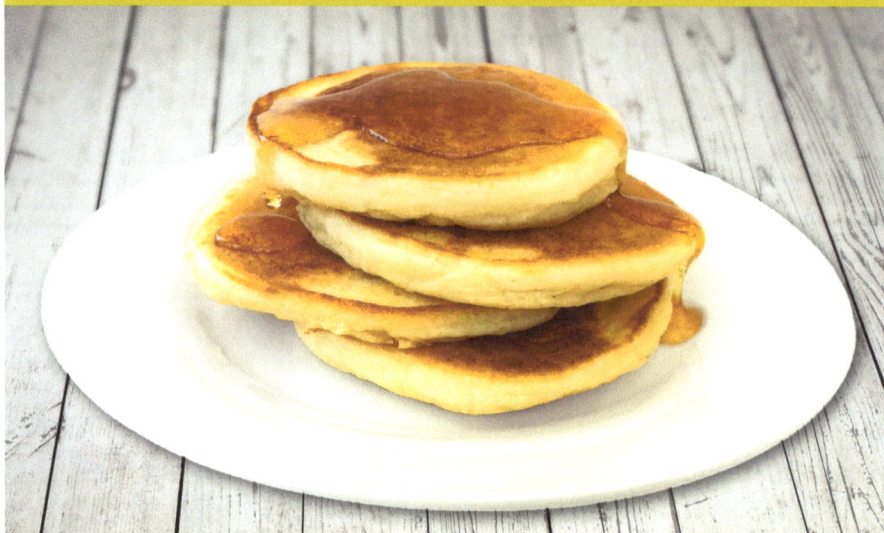

Ingredients

1 cup (250ml) gluten and wheat free self-raising flour ·
1 heaped tbsp. coconut flour · 1 tsp. healthy baking
powder · 2 tbsp. clear olive oil or liquid coconut oil ·
½ tsp. vanilla essence · 2 tbsp. rice malt syrup · ½ tsp.
fresh lemon juice · 1 egg · 200-250 ml almond milk · Pinch
of salt · Cinnamon to taste

Prep 20 min

Cook 20 min

2 Servings

Method:

1. Sift the gluten and wheat free self-raising flour, coconut flour, baking powder, and salt in a glass bowl.

2. Break the egg into a small bowl and add the vanilla essence, lemon juice, rice malt syrup, coconut oil or olive oil, and 200 ml almond milk. Mix well and pour into the dry ingredients.

3. Mix the dry ingredients and liquids well and add the rest of the almond milk (50ml) if needed to achieve desired batter thickness.

4. Use a large stick free pan and add a few drops of olive oil to the base of the pan. Heat up on a low-to-medium heat. Use a large spoon to pour the batter into three little pancakes. When the top of the batter becomes drier, turn the pancakes and bake the other side. When done transfer to a plate. Pour a few drops of olive oil again on the base of the pan and start baking the next three little pancakes.

5. When done, serve with rice malt syrup and cinnamon.

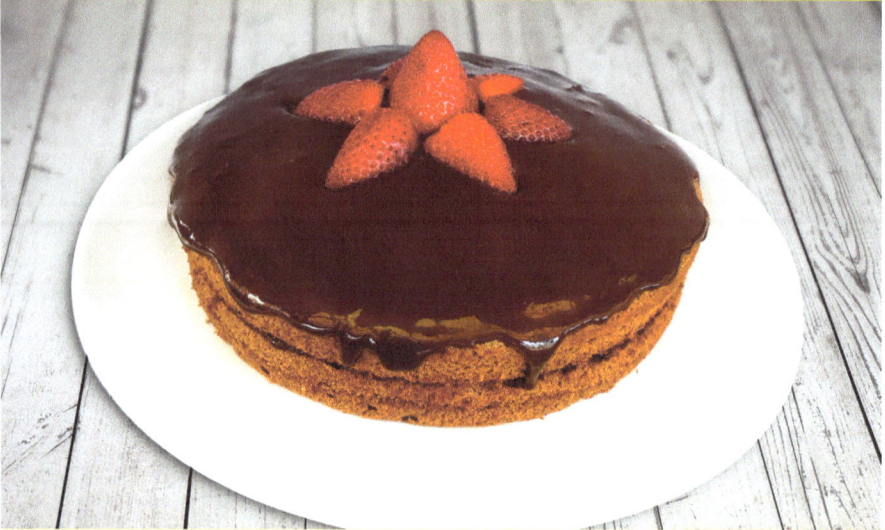

Healthy Chocolate Sponge Cake

Ingredients

250 ml gluten and wheat free self-raising flour · 50 ml Coconut flour · 3 eggs, separated · 1 tsp. vanilla essence · 50 ml olive oil or liquid coconut oil · ½ cup coconut sugar · ½ Cup (125 ml) of rice malt syrup · Pinch of salt · 4 tbsp. organic cacao mixed with 125 ml warm water · 2 round baking dishes (18cm in diameter) · 2 tsp. baking powder with clean ingredients and aluminium free · Olive oil baking spray

Prep 20 min

Cook 20 min

8 Servings

Method:

1. Turn on your fan forced oven and set it to 180 degree Celsius.

2. Sift flours, baking powder and salt into a glass bowl.

3. In another glass bowl mix the 3 egg yolks, coconut sugar, vanilla essence, coconut oil, rice malt syrup, honey, cacao with water.

4. Add all dry ingredients now with the wet mixture and mix till all ingredients are wet and creamy.

5. Whisk the egg whites till spongy and fold it lightly into the creamy chocolate batter mixture.

6. Spray the two round aluminium baking dishes and transfer the mixture into equal parts in each baking dish.

7. Bake for 15-20 minutes. After 15 minutes, test the cake in the centre quickly by inserting a thin blade pointy knife or tester stick, to see if it is cooked. Cake needs to be moist and not dry, as it still cooks a bit after you have removed it from the oven. Take it out of the oven when the knife point is clear from any raw batter.

8. After removing from the oven let it cool down for 5 min on a cooling down rack. Then remove from the baking dishes to stop further cooking and let it cool down for a further 15-20 minutes before icing.

Healthy Chocolate Icing Ingredients

Ingredients

¾ cup unsweetened cacao powder, sifted if there are lumps ▪ ¼ cup melted coconut oil ▪ ¼ - ½ cup of rice malt syrup ▪ 2-4 tbsp. honey or maple syrup (depending on your taste buds) ▪ 1 tsp. vanilla essence ▪ Splash of unsweetened almond milk (optional)

Icing Prep 20 min

Method:

1. Add all ingredients to a small mixing bowl. Mix until everything comes together and you have a thick, rich icing-like consistency.

2. Add a little more maple syrup/honey if it's not sweet enough or more cacao powder if the mixture is too runny.

3. Stir in a splash of almond milk if you find the consistency to be too thick.

4. Wait for the icing to cool down a bit when the coconut oil hardens, before spreading onto the cakes. Turn the one cake upside down on a plate, and spread some icing over before putting the other cake on top of it. Now spread a thicker layer of icing on the top of the cake. You can add a garnish like strawberries on top.

Tip: When the cake has cooled down over night, place it in the microwave for 5-10 seconds to warm it up and it will taste like a freshly baked cake.

Healthier Pizza Base

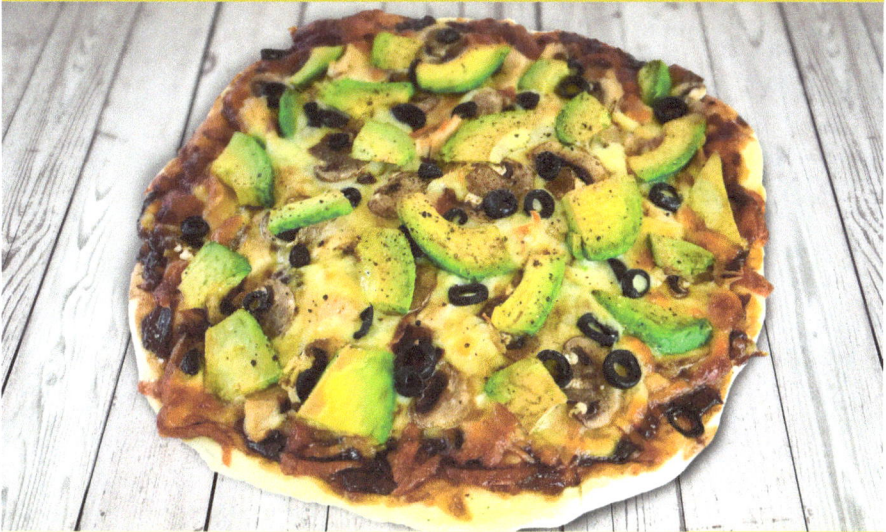

Ingredients

2 cups (500 ml) gluten and wheat free bread flour (if you cannot find gluten and wheat free bread flour, try normal flour) · 3 heaped tablespoons of coconut flour · ½ tsp. salt · 15 ml olive oil · 10 grams dried yeast · 200 ml lukewarm water

Pizza Base
Prep 15 min
Rising 1 hour

Pizza Topping and baking 30 min

2-4 Servings

Method:

1. Mix all ingredients well and place in a glass bowl.

2. Cover the bowl with cling wrap and place it on top of a tea towel. Then cover with two more tea towels to keep the heat in for a bit longer. This will help the dough rise nicely.

3. Let it rise for an hour before making the pizza base on baking paper.

Pizza Topping

(Spread the following ingredients evenly over the pizza base)

Ingredients

Caramelised onion, barbecue sauce or tomato sauce · Cup full of mozzarella cheese · 2-3 thin rings of onion · 3-4 medium size mushrooms · Cup full of cooked shredded chicken strips or fried mincemeat · One avocado · ½ cup of olives · Salt and pepper to taste

Prep 15 min

Method:

Bake for 18-20 minutes in a 180 degree Celsius fan forced oven.

Omelette

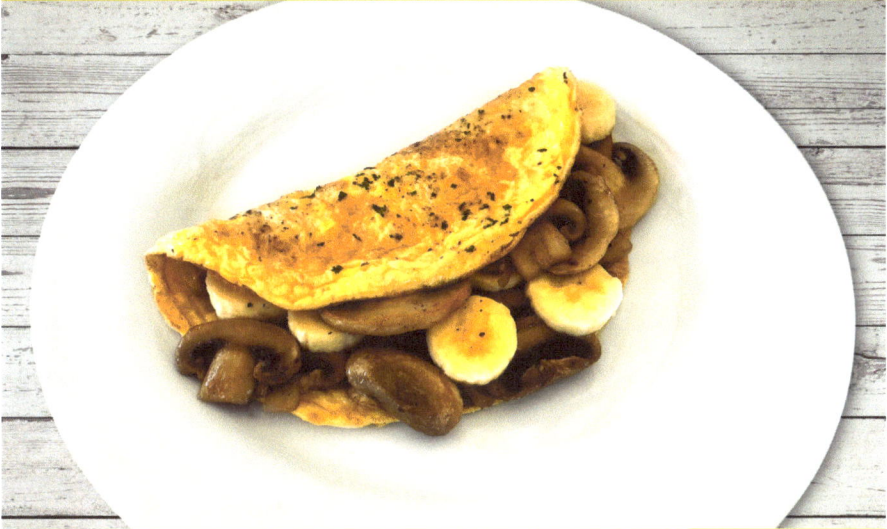

Ingredients

2 eggs · 2 tbsp. water · 2 medium size mushrooms sliced · 2 rings of onion · 1 small to medium banana · 1 tbsp. grass-fed butter · 1 tbsp. olive oil

Prep 10 min

Cook 10 min

1 Serving

Method:

1. Fry the onion rings and sliced mushrooms in the olive oil in a small pan and remove from the heat when done.

2. Mix the eggs and water in a small bowl, now melt the grass-fed butter in a medium pan over low-to-medium heat and pour the egg mixture in the pan.

3. Add salt and pepper to taste.

4. When the one side is cooked, turn the omelette around in the pan.

5. Remove from the heat and add the mushroom and onion mixture on the one half of the omelette. Cut the banana in wheels on this same half, and close the omelette.

6. Lift it out of the pan and serve.

Maize Meal Porridge

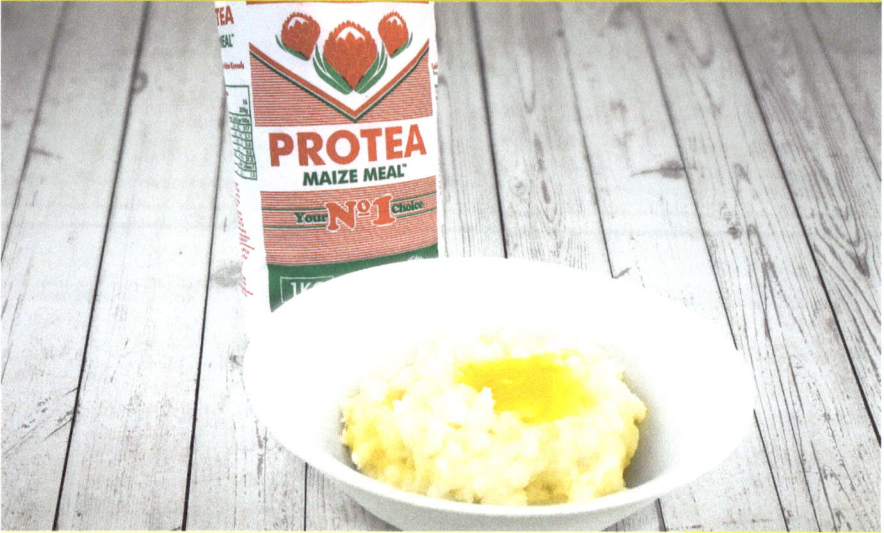

Ingredients

1 cup (250 ml) maize meal porridge · ½ tsp. salt · 1 tsp. grass-fed butter · 750 ml of boiling water

Prep 10 min

Cook
15-20 min

2 Servings

This is an Africa dish and if you cannot find it in the normal supermarket, you'll find it at a South African market. You can even use the Italian version called Polenta if you are more familiar with that one.

Method:

1. Sift the maize meal.

2. Bring the water, grass-fed butter, and salt to the boil.

3. Turn the heat down to low. Remove the pot for a minute and add the maize meal to the water. Then stir well with a fork.

4. Place back on the low heat stove plate and close the lid of the pot. Stir every 5 minutes. Cook for 15-20 minutes and remove from the heat.

You can eat this porridge with a teaspoon of grass-fed butter, 2 teaspoons of coconut sugar, and unsweetened almond milk. Or you can keep it a savoury dish and serve with the following toppings

Option 1

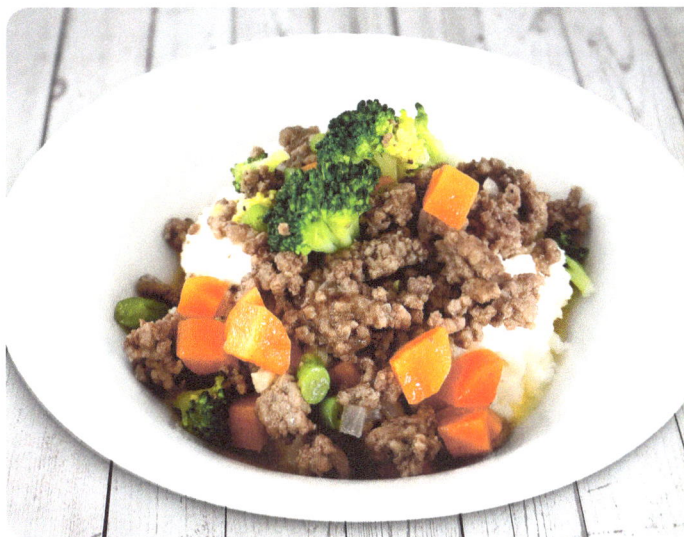

Prep 10 min
Cook 15 min
1 Serving

Fry 250 grams of mincemeat. When halfway cooked, add the following veggies: 1 medium carrot cut into cubes, 4 broccoli pieces cut in smaller pieces, 8 small green beans cut up small. Add a half cup of water and cook on high for 3-5 minutes, or till water is gone. Veggies must still be a bit crunchy. At the end of the cooking add one teaspoon of gluten and wheat free gravy powder mixed with a half cup of water and cook on high for 3 minutes. Serve this meat dish on top of the maize meal porridge.

Option 2

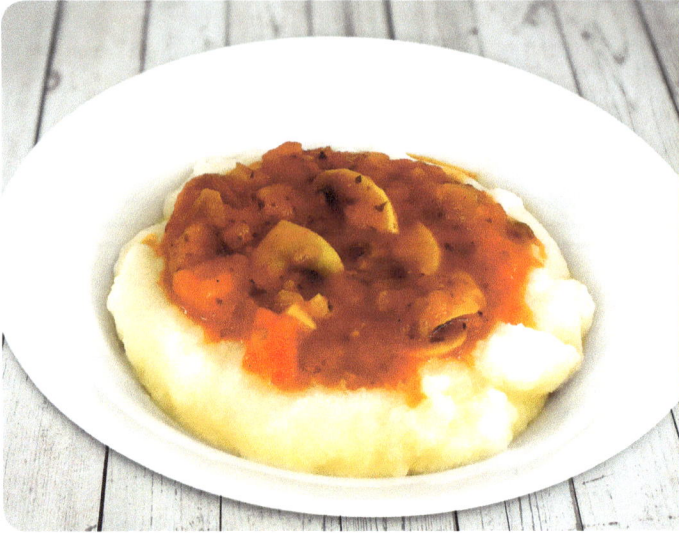

Prep 10 min
Cook 15 min
1 Serving

Fry a small onion, and 3 medium size mushrooms sliced.
Add two peeled diced tomatoes and half cup of water.
Add salt, pepper, and curry to taste. Cook for 10-15 minutes.
Serve on top of the maize meal porridge.

Option 3

Beef sausage and gravy sauce. Serve the sausage next to the maize meal porridge and the gravy sauce on top.

NATURAL REMEDIES FOR EVERYDAY AILMENTS

Do everything in your power to heal your family and your aches a natural way, to avoid any possible side effects from medications, without being ignorant or worsening your suffering by not reading the signs right. Never experiment on your babies or children with health remedies when they cannot really tell you how they feel, as this can be fatal. It is always wise to take your child to a doctor to make sure they are not at risk of something sinister. Depending on what is wrong with your child, you can always discuss with your doctor then. You can say you'd rather they recommend something more natural. If there is nothing natural that will work for the specific condition, just go with what the doctor prescribes because they usually know better. For the normal aches that come every now and then, the following techniques are how I treat myself naturally.

Headache

Drink one or two cups of green tea. If you cannot get used to the strong aftertaste of the green tea, add a teaspoon of honey. Then take ten to twenty deep breaths while trying to relax your muscles. You can also put an ice pack on your neck and shoulders for a bit. Or, take a walk for 20 minutes to relax your muscles and get some oxygen into your veins by breathing deeply. This is what I usually do, and my headache disappears within 20-30 minutes. Common causes of headaches are work stress, neck strain for sitting in the same position for long periods, not enough oxygen, hunger, cold and flu symptoms, lack of sleep, or unhealthy eating habits.

Nausea

Ginger is an effective natural remedy to treat nausea. Peel a small piece of fresh ginger and cut into small cubes. Put it in a small teapot with a strainer. Pour hot water over the ginger cubes and let it stand for a few minutes to cool down, before drinking a small glass to get rid of your nausea.

BLOATING

Consume probiotics (good bacteria) daily. This will help you get rid of the uncomfortable feeling of bloating. Food probiotics are found in natural yogurt, kefir, which is a fermented probiotic milk drink, and kombucha, which is a fermented black or green tea. You can also buy a probiotic supplement from the pharmacy or health food store, and take a tablet per day to prevent any bloating. Peppermint tea also helps with bloating. If your bloating is chronic, it may be time to make a change to your overall diet as discussed in this book.

INFLAMMATION AND/OR WARM FEELING IN THE BACK AND NECK

Exercising and moving regularly is the best way to get rid of aches in the back and neck caused by inflammation. You'll have to get the blood circulating and also inhale deeply for the oxygen to spread to all cells in the body. Increased blood circulation takes oxygen and nutrition to the cells, and also removes toxins through the lymphatic system. The lymphatic system is a network of tissues and organs that help rid the body of toxins, waste and other unwanted materials. The primary function of the lymphatic system is to transport lymph, a fluid containing infection-fighting white blood cells, throughout the body. Unlike blood, which flows throughout the body in a continues loop, lymph flows in only one direction, upward toward the neck. Since the lymphatic system does not have a heart to pump it, its upward movement depends on the motions of the muscle and joint pumps achieved through movement of the body. The lymph fluid transports through larger lymphatic vessels to lymph nodes, where it is cleaned by lymphocytes, before emptying ultimately into the right or the left subclavian veins located below the clavicles at the base of the neck, where it mixes back with the blood. Go for a quick walk or cycling every day for 30 minutes and drink at least six glasses of water.

Alternatively, what I use is ice packs at the back of my neck and the soft tissue of my shoulders to calm down any inflammation or the uncomfortable warm feeling. For continued aches and inflammation in your back and neck, book a consultation session at your doctor or chiropractor to make sure it is only the normal every day wear and tear, and not anything else to worry about.

BACK PAIN AND STIFFNESS

Use a tennis ball and stand against a wall. Now push the tennis ball in between your back and the wall so that you have a good grip on it that it does not fall to the ground easily. Now move left to right, and up and down, so that the tennis ball rolls on the soft tissue next to the spine, lower back, and the shoulders. Move the tennis ball regularly to the targeted spots on your back and shoulders. It will help the muscles to relax. This is the closest you can get for giving yourself a back massage. You can even use the tennis ball as a pressure point on the knots in your back to release and relax it. Muscles stick together and create knots because of inactivity, dehydration, and injury. When muscle fibres start to stick to each other and become adhered, this new hard and lumpy feeling is a 'muscle knot'. When we sit in front of a computer all day long in the same position, we lose our flexibility and create knots. So again, regular movement, drinking adequate fluids per day, and eating a healthy diet will help prevent muscle knots.

STOMACH CRAMPS AND DIARRHOEA

It is important to stay hydrated when you are experiencing abdominal pain and diarrhoea. Drink plenty of clear liquids, such as water, tea, juice, and broth.

For any severe and chronic aches and pains, go and see your general practitioner to run a few tests to check what the underlying problem is.

THE TRUTHS ABOUT FACE AND NECK EXERCISES

It was 1990 and the final or third year of me studying *Beauty Technology* in South Africa. I had done an assignment on face and neck exercises. I still have this in my possession after all these years. Those years these exercises were not well known amongst the public. Today if you Google them, you'll find multiple websites offering face exercise programs and books. I'll be honest and say that over all these years I have not done regular face and neck exercises as I probably should have. But I did realise when I looked at this assignment during 2017 that there were a few of the exercises that must have stuck in my head from doing the assignment, which I unknowingly did over the years. They were some neck stretches and cheek stretches.

For a few months I have been testing some of these face exercises to see if they can tighten the muscles in my face. And by the middle of March 2018, I could see a slight change around my eyes in the small time frame I have tested them. I'll also admit that I've had three Botox injection sessions in my face before, and one filler between my eyes over the past six years. Therefore I am familiar with what can be achieved with these facial rejuvenation treatments. At present my last Botox injections were two years ago. I strongly believe that you must give your face a break and make sure that the muscles are tightening and learning to work again in between Botox treatments.

For these treatments, I visited two experienced doctors. You really must not try to get away with the cheapest wrinkle-relaxer injections, because you might get them administered by a person that is not fully qualified or experienced. I, for sure, do not want to be anyone's guinea pig to help them gain their experience. When wrinkle-relaxers and fillers are not administered the right way, a person can look fake and malformed. The reason why I talk about a wrinkle-relaxer at the start of this face and neck exercises section, is to compare the different results, and give you the full truth as I have experienced it, as well as from the researcher's point of view.

With a wrinkle-relaxer and filler you'll get an instantly younger appearance. By instant I mean after you get wrinkle-relaxer injections in your forehead and 'crow's feet' (which are the laughing wrinkles at the sides of the eyes), it takes between 3-10 days for the wrinkle-relaxer to settle and work through the muscles to paralyse them, keeping them from working for the next three months. My experience was that it took 14-21 days after I received the injections for my face to start looking smooth and relaxed. After three months the Botox will gradually work out and this will slowly bring movement back to the muscles. My results lasted about 5-6 months. The muscles usually are now weakened and not as strong as when you first got the wrinkle-relaxer injected. And of course it is not inexpensive to get a wrinkle-relaxer treatment, especially at a qualified and experienced professional.

My advice is when you want to get treatments to change your appearance, either temporarily or permanently, is that you must visit professionals and be willing to pay for their experience. If your budget does not allow this, save a bit longer or make use of other more natural ways to look younger. It works the same as when a woman wants to get breast implants. For this kind of cosmetic procedure you deserve to visit the best cosmetic surgeon with a good track record, because you do not want any mistakes as a result of such a big decision. The same rule applies here: you should want to do it for you, and not for someone else. If your focus changes from you to others, you may be deeply disappointed after you have made a permanent change to your body.

When it comes to face and neck exercises, it takes years of regular exercises to make a huge improvement in a face to look younger, but they can easily take off five to ten years from your real age. They do not cost anything except for using your determination and exercising regularly. The sooner that one starts with these exercises in life, the better the results will be when you get to your forties and fifties. To successfully pull off the face and neck exercise regime and look younger, you must combine them with a good daily cleansing routine as I have detailed in the first part of this book. The other two important factors are protecting your skin from sun damage and being on a healthy diet as explained in the *Building blocks for good and healthy skin* section. Although face and neck exercises will have a good impact and make you look younger, they can never create as dramatic an effect as a wrinkle-relaxer and filler. What face and neck exercises will do for you is to help you age gracefully. Aging gracefully needs to be our focus, and not trying to stay young forever. As long as you keep this in mind, you'll be happier and more confident in life.

Face and neck exercises cannot do any harm if done correctly. Think about it this way: just as a person can hurt themselves from doing an exercise the wrong way in the gym, or doing it too many times, we can hurt ourselves the same way with face and neck exercises. Do not jump straight into an exercise that someone tells you to do. Make sure they are safe and not creating more wrinkles, or stretching the skin too much. Listen to qualified and experienced trainers.

It is never too early to start these exercises. Young women in their early twenties can use the face and neck exercises to prevent lines and sagging skin from forming. To keep the face and neck firmer and smoother, you'll have to schedule regular exercise sessions during the week. The question that most people ask is 'How soon will I see results when I start with face and neck exercises?' The answer is 'It depends on each individual'. Determinant factors are: age, skin damage, regularity of the exercises, how well you perform the exercises, daily skin practices, and diet. Regardless of age, you will still achieve results by doing regular face and neck exercises, but the younger the skin, the quicker the results because the skin is still firm and elastic.

Facial shape is the determinant factor of attractiveness, and particularly facial symmetry. The bones that you were born with give your face its unique shape and structure. Generally speaking, the only way that you can change the shape of your facial bones is through cosmetic surgery. I vote for being happy with who we are and making ourselves look attractive and beautiful through the correct skin care treatments, grooming, and styling techniques. Why would you want to go to extremes to change who you are? There is not another YOU on this planet. (Except for someone who may resemble you, called your double because your looks are quite similar, or your identical twin. But the fact is that there will still be huge differences.) Celebrate your uniqueness! Instead, spend your money on learning how to groom yourself, caring for your hands and feet, investing in a lifestyle of healthy eating and exercise, looking after your skin in order to stay younger for longer, getting a hairstyle that fits your features, and learning the tricks of how you can look amazing through the use of the correct clothing styles and colours for you. My book *Style Yourself with Confidence* is an easy way that women can learn how to dress their body shape and features best.

Another mistake that some people make is to think someone else is more beautiful than them, whereas that same person may think the other way around, and think you are more beautiful. You see the truth is that 'beauty is in the eye of the beholder'. So what may be beautiful and attractive for you, may not be the same for someone else. When you start to celebrate who you are, you'll come to the point where you accept yourself, and your life will be more enjoyable.

Let's be honest with ourselves though! For example: if you are overweight and not loving the way you look, start doing something about it. Do not sit all day long and keep eating to the point where you feel sick. Stop with those bad habits and start being determined that you can change your life around. Soon afterwards, you'll reap the wonderful benefits of addressing your obstacles. Change usually starts when we are honest with ourselves.

FACE EXERCISES

There are six things to remember when it comes to face and neck exercises. Firstly, do not perform an exercise that creates wrinkles. Wrinkles originate from repetitive facial movements for example frowning a lot. Decades ago when face exercises was introduced, some exercises created wrinkles while performing it. Over the past decade or so they realised it is no use in doing exercises for the face that creates wrinkles, because the repetitive movements increased and deepened the wrinkles.

So when you choose a face exercise program, make sure the exercises do not create any wrinkles. As soon as you start with my face exercises, you'll understand what I mean. Secondly, do not stretch the skin with your hands or fingers, but rather support the skin during an exercise through pressure points. Regular stretching of the skin causes wrinkles and small tears in the skin. Thirdly, breathe well during the exercise session because smooth and efficient breathing is crucial for delivering the oxygen to the areas that need to perform the exercise properly. Fourth, before starting with the exercises, cleanse the skin, then apply a layer of natural oil over the face and neck such as olive oil, coconut oil, jojoba oil, almond oil, tissue oil, or even a thick layer of moisturiser will work. The oil will make the skin supple and prevent damage through possible stretching. It works the same when a woman is pregnant and her tummy stretches out of proportion to accommodate the baby inside. But applying a rich layer of olive oil over the whole tummy area after each shower prevents any stretch marks in the skin. This trick was passed on to me by my mother, and although I have a small build, I carried two daughters and have zero stretch marks. The oil on the face and neck during each exercise session will provide the same protection. Fifth, start with facial and neck warming-up exercises before going into the real exercises. Sixth, always do your face and neck exercises in front of a mirror so that you can see if you are doing it the correct way, and that the muscles are working in such a way that you do not create more wrinkles. By looking at your reflection, you'll also notice when you are stretching the skin, rather than using pressure points to stop the other muscles from contracting and creating wrinkles.

The basic rules while doing the exercises are as follows:

1. Your starting position should be with a good posture. If you are sitting or standing, keep your head up straight, shoulders relaxed and no slouching or leaning forward.

2. Work slowly towards tightening the muscle while keeping the skin firm with your fingers, holding for a bit, and releasing slowly again. Slowly movements are the key here.

3. When you are doing the face exercises correctly, there should be no wrinkles or loose skin between the corners of the eyes and your hairline. Even the forehead must make no wrinkles when performing an exercise.

4. Choose a time during the day when you can relax and will not be disturbed. Sit quietly and relaxed while breathing deeply for a minute or two. Close your eyes, breathe in and hold for one count, and breathe out and hold for one count. Repeat this breathing for 1-2 minutes and feel how the tension releases from all the muscles in your body.

5. Exercise the face and neck muscles for 15 minutes every day or for 30 minutes, four times per week.

Depending on the time of day when you do your face and neck exercises, you can get rid of the extra oil on the skin after the exercise session by blotting the skin with a facial tissue. Doing your face and neck exercises during the evening, you can leave the rest of the oil on the skin serving as a moisturiser. When you still need to apply make-up afterwards, cleanse the face and neck as usual with your face cleanser, following with the normal steps of toning and moisturising.

Oily and problem skin types should always cleanse the face afterwards to remove the oil, as the extra oil can irritate or inflame the skin further. Rather use an essential oil that has an anti-inflammatory effect on the skin like bergamot, eucalyptus, rose, fennel, or thyme. Any person with a problem skin who uses prescription medications or creams must always check with their dermatologist first to see if they can use any other oil or product with their current prescriptions. This is a precaution to take so that your skin will not flare up again.

Face and neck exercises improve blood circulation, giving your skin a healthy colour. The correct procedure in doing your exercises is to *tighten the muscles slowly, hold, and then release slowly.* Controlling the release is as important as tightening and holding. Not doing it this way, may make your exercises useless that will have no impact on what you are trying to achieve.

Easy ways to know if your face and neck exercises are working well are if someone asks you if you were on a holiday, because you look so healthy and relaxed. If you are a woman wearing make-up they may ask you if you changed your make-up because you look so different. Other positive comments may come your way like: 'You look beautiful,' for the ladies, or 'handsome' for the guys. Or 'You look so fresh today'.

The muscles of the face are unique compared to the muscles in the body. While most muscles in the body connect to and move only bones, facial muscles mostly connect to bones and the skin. Science says there are forty-three muscles in the face. Following are face and neck exercises with photos to explain it better. Can guys also do it, or is it only for the ladies? These exercises are for all adults, and guys will benefit from doing it as well.

The following is an image of the muscles seen from the front:

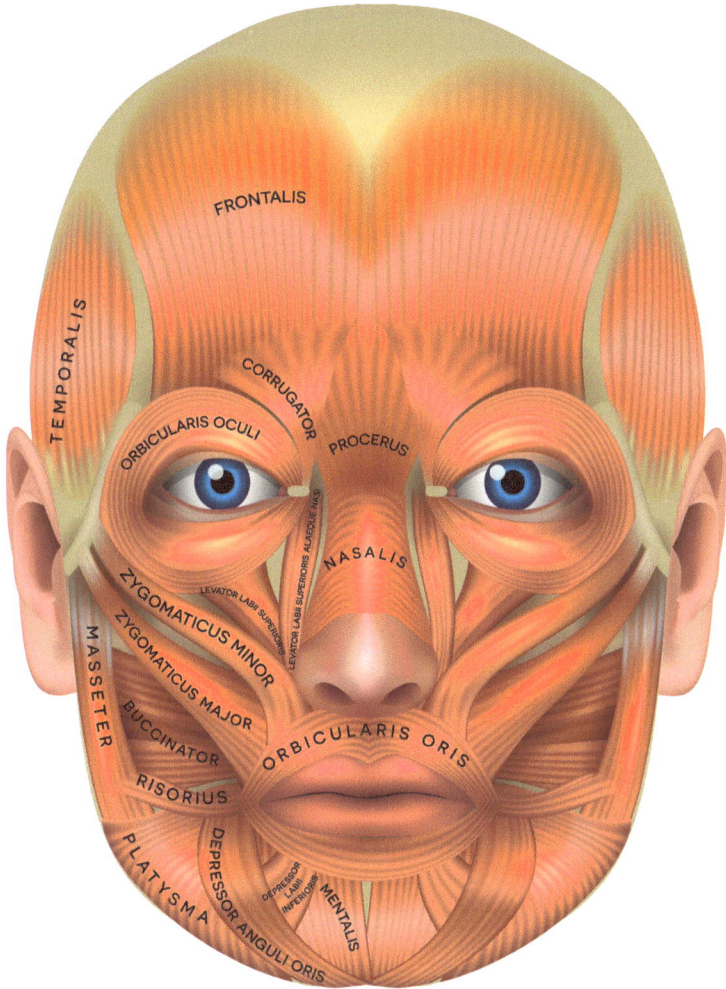

Muscles of the face from the front

Neck exercises

The correct neck exercises can help you release tension, stiffness, tightness, reduce pain, and increase flexibility. A strong neck can also help prevent neck and cervical injuries. Overworking and misusing of the muscles in the neck can lead to pain or injuries. When you exercise the neck, take care not to stress or strain your neck. Use slow, controlled movements to complete the exercises. You do not have to exercise your neck every day, give a day or two to rest in between. Go at your own pace and take it slow when you start. You can increase the intensity and duration of your neck exercises as you progress. If you have chronic neck pain, speak to your doctor first, before starting with a neck exercise program.

A good face and neck exercise routine

A 30 minute routine for four times per week or a 15 minute routine every day. (For a 15 minute routine cut the repeats in the below program in half).

Warm-up exercises for the neck

1. **Cleanse the face and neck and apply an oil or cream all over**. Make sure all the skin is covered, but do not overuse the product.

2. **Sit quietly and relax while breathing deeply for a minute or two**. Close your eyes, breathe in and hold for one count, breathe out and hold for one count. Feel the tension release from all the muscles in your body.

3. Sit or stand in front of a mirror now.

   Sit up straight, **drop your chin to your chest** and hold for two counts, bring the head back in position facing directly ahead, then push the head backwards to the back and hold for two counts, while keeping your jaw relaxed, and breathing deeply throughout.

   Repeat each movement for four times. In total you will do each movement for five times.

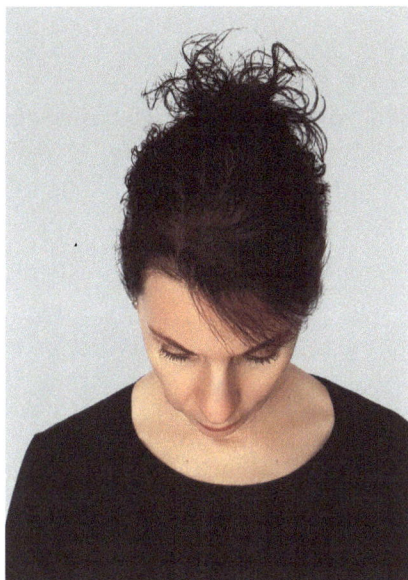

4. Turn your head from side to side to look over your shoulders. **Look to the right** and hold for two counts, bring the head back in position facing directly ahead, then **look to the left** and hold for two counts. Repeat four times for each movement. In total you will do each movement five times. Do not force the muscles while you are doing it. The movements should be gentle.

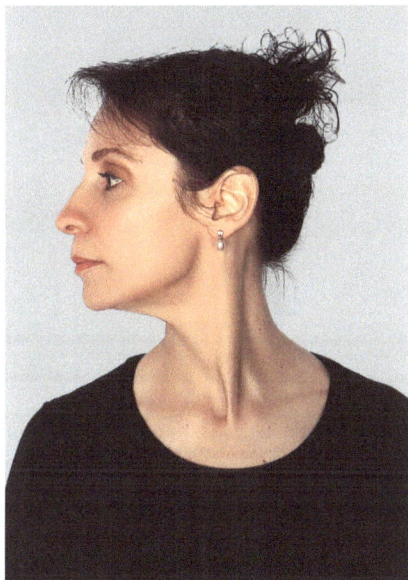

5. Drop your chin to your chest and **roll the head from left to right doing a half circle**. Roll your chin to the right and hold for two counts, then roll to the left and hold for two counts.

Repeat each movement four times. In total you will do each movement five times.

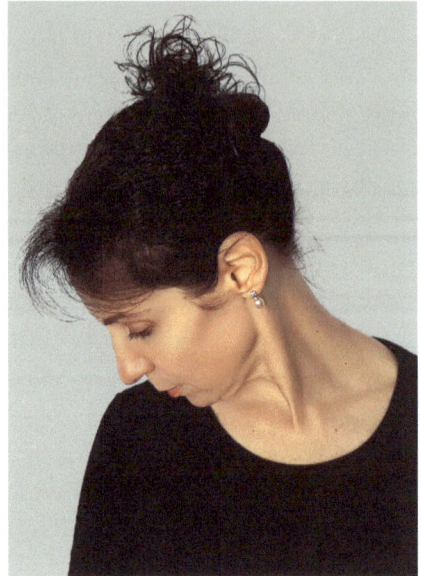

6. Keep your chin dropped to your chest and **roll the head now in a full circle**, starting at the front. Roll the head around as if you want to touch the back of the shoulders. Do not force the head to accidently pull a muscle. They must be gentle and relaxed circles.

Roll the head slowly five times to the left and then five times to the right. If you feel any pain at the back of the neck while doing this exercise, stop it immediately and move on to the next exercise. This exercise is safer to do while you are sitting or holding onto something so that you do not lose your balance and fall over.

Neck stretches

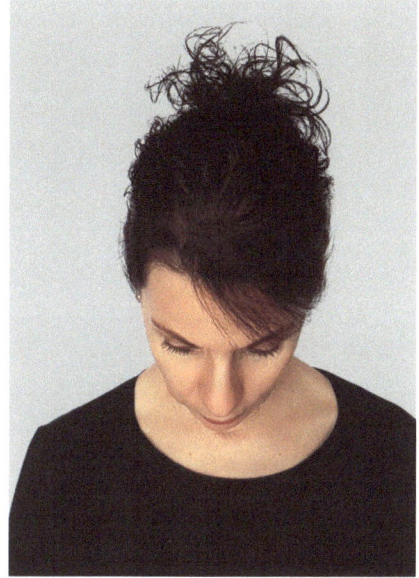

1. **Slowly drop your head forward** so that your chin almost touches your chest, and **hold for ten counts**. Feel the stretch at the back of your neck. Bring your head slowly back to position facing directly ahead, before the next stretch.

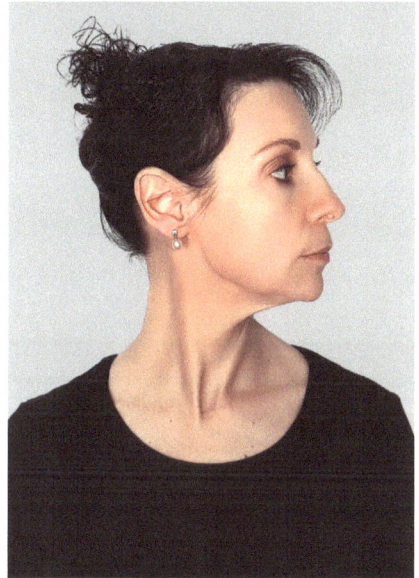

2. Slowly turn your head to **look over your left shoulder, and hold for ten counts**. Feel the stretch under your chin and down your throat. Bring your head slowly back to position facing directly ahead, before the next stretch.

3. Slowly turn your head to **look over your right shoulder, and hold for ten counts**. Feel the stretch under your chin and down your throat. Bring your head slowly back to position facing directly ahead, before the next stretch.

4. **Gently drop your head backwards, open your mouth wide, and hold for ten counts.** Feel the stretch under your chin and down your throat. Bring your head slowly back to position facing directly ahead, before the next stretch.

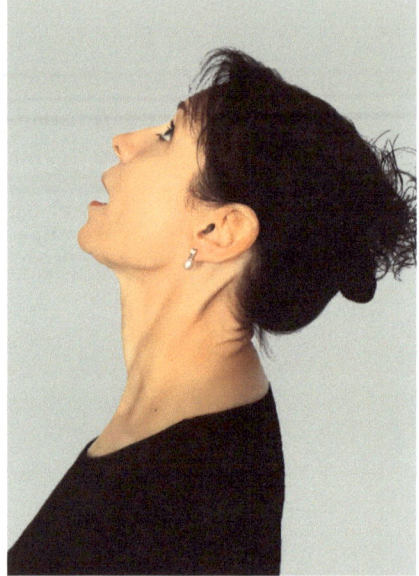

5. **Look diagonally up to the left and hold for ten counts.** Feel the stretch from under your chin and down the side of the neck. Bring your head slowly back to position facing directly ahead, before the next stretch.

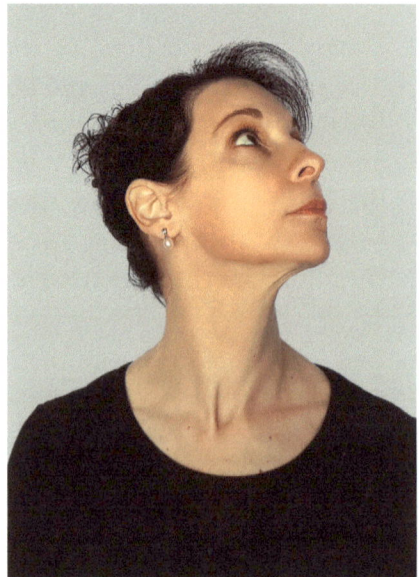

6. Now **look diagonally down to the right and hold for ten counts** before slowly releasing and returning to position. Feel the stretch under the chin, on the back and the sides of the neck. Return to position facing directly ahead before the next stretch.

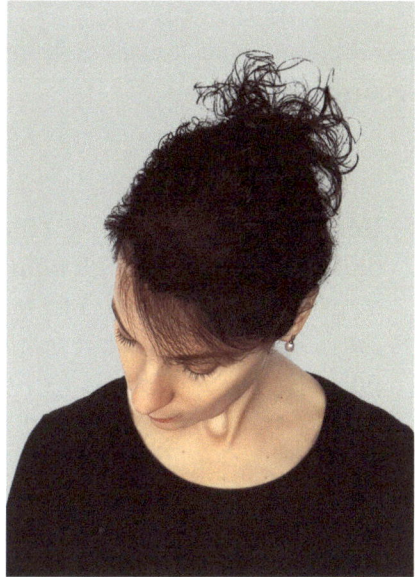

7. **Look diagonally up to the right and hold for ten counts.** Return to position.

8. **Look diagonally down to the left and hold for ten counts**. Return to position.

Face warm-up exercises
For these exercises look straight in the mirror to make sure you are doing it correctly.

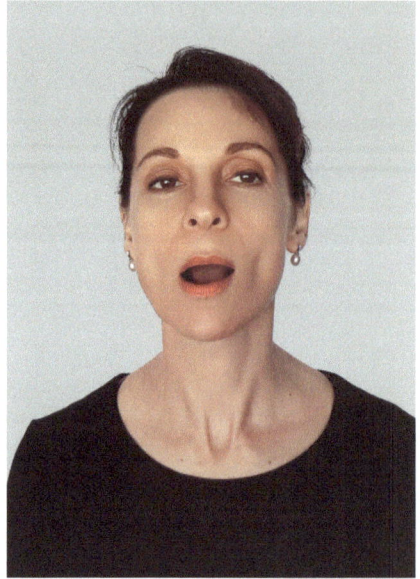

1. **Imagine you are chewing a huge ball of gum, without clenching or grinding the teeth.** You basically chew the air in your mouth, pulling your face cheeks to the left and then to the right. Pulling your lips up and down, and to the sides. Pull the funny faces without creating many wrinkles in the face. Do these warming-up exercises quickly for 30 seconds to 1 minute.

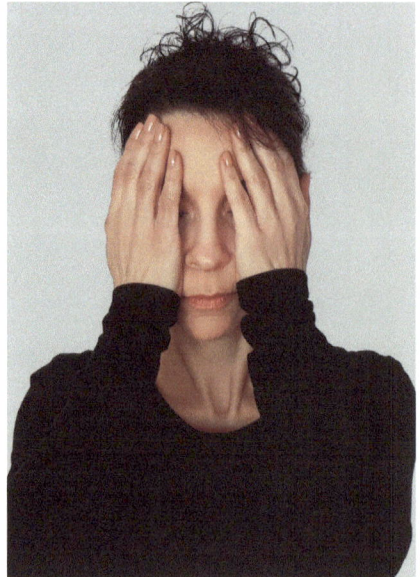

2. **Rub your hands together to warm them up.** Close your eyes and place your warm hands **over the sides of your face**, then hold them for ten counts to warm-up the face. Repeat another two times.

3. **Pour 5-6 drops of face oil in one hand**. Now rub the oil between your fingers warming-up the oil. Use your fingers to apply the oil on your cheeks and forehead in gentle upwards motions. Use only your fingers now to **massage the left cheek upwards with ten strokes, then go to your right cheek and massage upwards with ten strokes.**

The technique for how you use your fingers is almost like a fan where you start with your left hand's fingers, starting with the forefinger, followed quickly with your middle finger, then your ring finger and pinkie; lifting the skin up gently with each finger. Follow with your right hand's fingers straight after you finished with the pinkie of the left hand. They are quick, but gentle upwards strokes with every finger following quickly after each other. Refrain from stretching the skin.

Finally go to your forehead and use your fingers to massage upwards from left to right with twenty strokes.

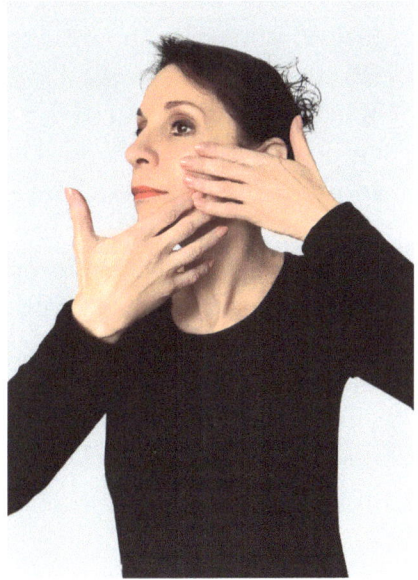

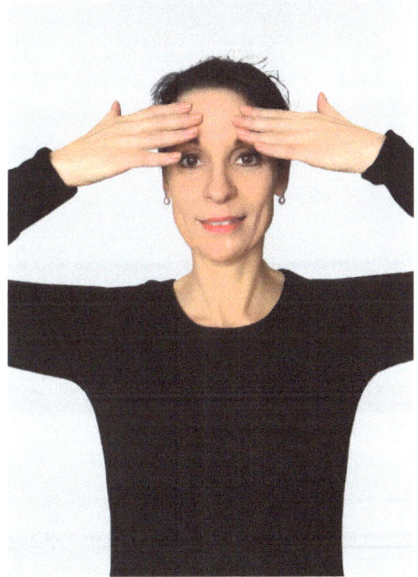

Cheek lifts

1. Face directly ahead and take a deep breath. While the lips are closed, **fill your mouth and cheeks with air**. Keep the lips tight so that the air does not escape. Hold the air in while **pulling the chin and jaw muscles up, and hold for ten counts**. Breathe slowly through your nose. Then slowly release the air through your lips and relax the cheeks for five counts.

   Repeat another two times so that you would have done three in total.

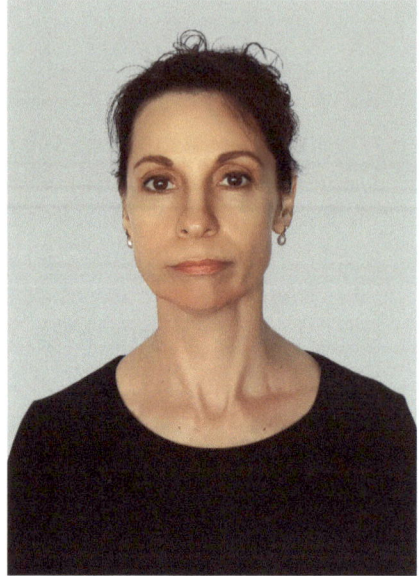

2. **Close your lips gently, smile slowly upwards without exposing your teeth, pulling the cheeks slowly upwards, and hold for ten counts**. Now slowly relax the cheeks.

   Repeat another three times so that you would have done four exercises in total. If your eyes wrinkle up on the sides, use your fingers gently to make pressure points on the skin, to stop it from wrinkling.

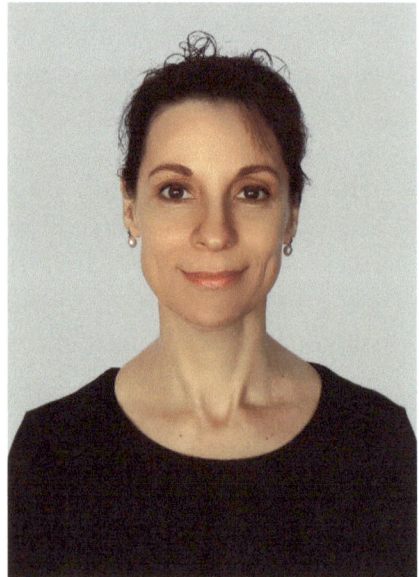

Eyebrow lifts

1. a) Stand in front of the mirror and place your four fingers of each hand over your forehead on each side. Use the fingers by pressing gently to prevent the skin from moving while you are doing the following exercise.

   b) Now pull up the eyebrows slowly and hold for one count. Repeat three times so that you do four quick lifts in total.

   c) Do the same exercise but this time **lift the eyebrows slowly and hold for ten counts before releasing slowly**. Repeat two times so that you do three in total.

2. Keep the same position in front of the mirror as the previous exercise and place your four fingers gently on each side of your forehead to keep the muscles from creating wrinkles. **Now frown as if you are trying to pull your eyebrows to meet in the middle, and hold for ten counts**. Release slowly and repeat another two times.

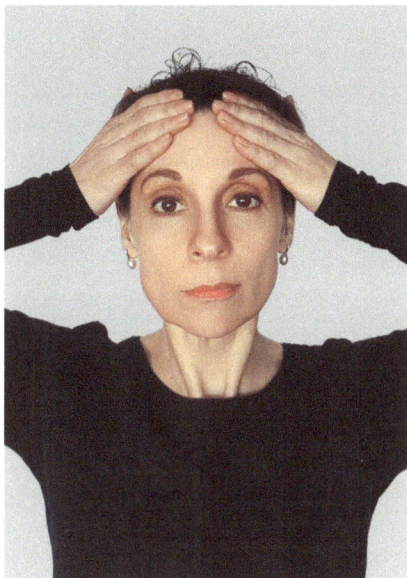

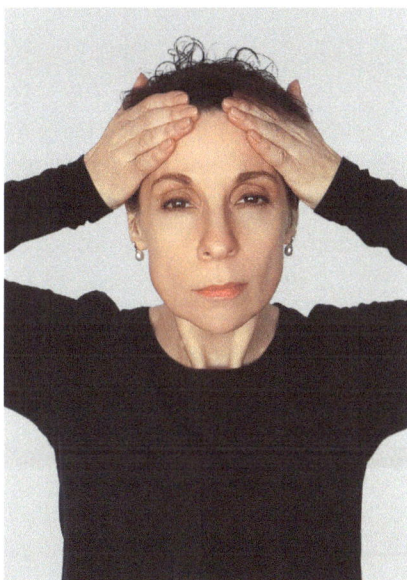

Lower eyelid lifts
This exercise is good for hollows and bags under the eyes.

1. Rub your hands together to warm the palms of your hands. **Close your eyes and place your warm palms gently over your eyes to warm them up**. Hold it for ten counts.

    Repeat this another two times.

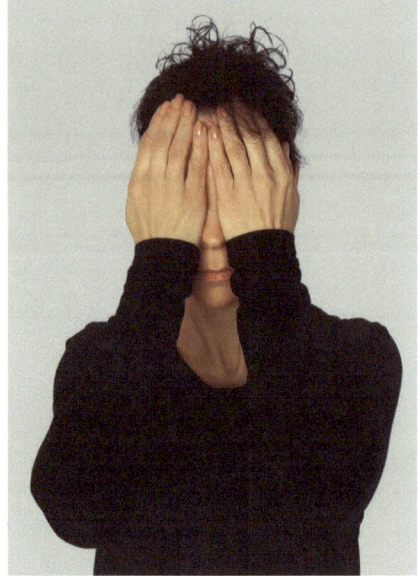

2. a) Stand in front of a mirror. **Take your three fingers (forefinger, middle finger and ring finger), and press the skin gently under the eyes** to prevent making wrinkles while doing the following exercise. Do not pull or stretch the skin while holding it in place. Also prevent your nails from digging into the skin. Use the soft parts of the finger tips to gently press and hold.

    b) **Open both eyes wide and hold for ten counts.** Then relax slowly.

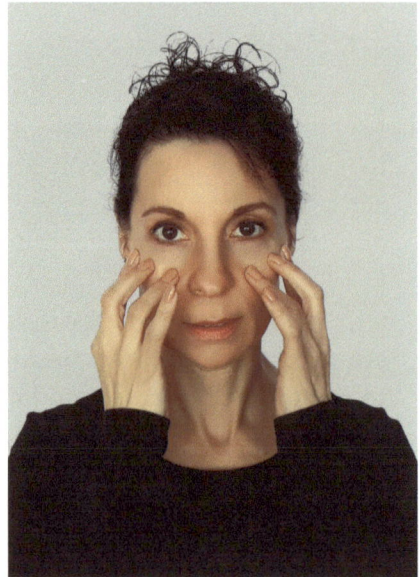

3. Keep the same position and **slowly pull up the lower eyelids and hold for ten counts**. Slowly release.

    Repeat another three times.

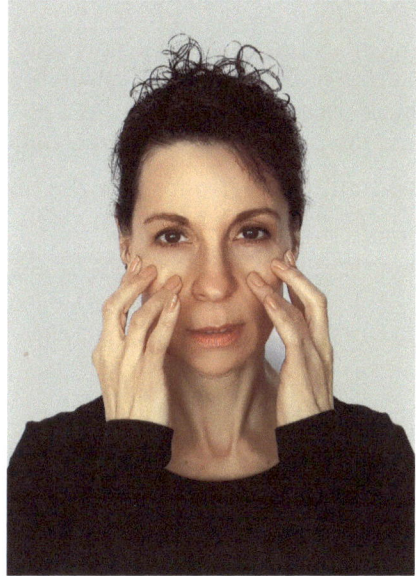

4. Rub your hands together again to warm the palms of your hands. **Close your eyes and place your warm palms over your closed eyes.** Relax the eyes and hold the hands over the eyes for ten to twenty counts. Repeat another one to two times.

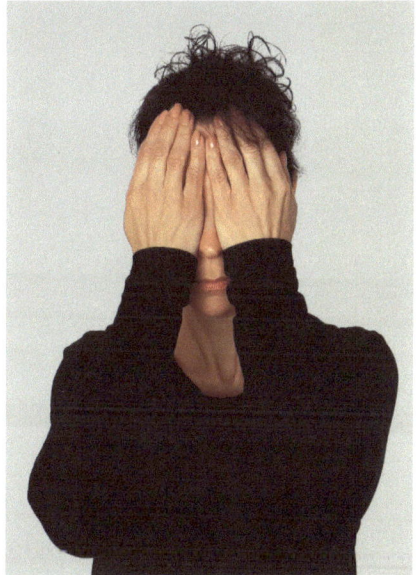

5. Finish by **sitting quietly and relaxed while breathing deeply for a minute or two**. Close your eyes, breathe in and hold for one count, breathe out and hold for one count. Feel the tension release from all the muscles in your body.

Congratulations, you have successfully completed your face and neck exercise routine!

Over time you will remember all these exercises in order and do it without having to look in the book.

BODY POSTURE

Our body posture is so important to our health and appearance that I have decided to include the information that I have written in my published book *Style Yourself with Confidence.*

Good posture helps keep bones and joints in the correct alignment so that muscles are used properly to avoid developing an abnormal permanent position. Proper posture also reduces abnormal wear and tear on joint surfaces, which can lead to arthritis. It decreases the stress on the ligaments holding the joints of the spine together, and preventing the spine from becoming fixed in an abnormal position. Good posture and back support are essential to avoid back and neck pain. It enhances proper breathing, ensuring oxygen and nutrients going to all the organs for optimal health and functioning.

When standing, stand up straight with your weight distributed evenly on both feet. Imagine a string running from your chest bone to the ceiling, suspending you like a marionette. Now drop your shoulders and shake your head slightly from side to side. You should now be standing correctly. Regularly practise standing this way in front of a mirror, and walk while pulling up through your midriff, head held high and shoulders down. Swing your legs from the joint at the hip rather than the knee when you walk. This way of walking is smooth and elegant.

You can definitely change your body posture through focusing on how you walk and sit every day. The time frame for developing a beautiful and upright body posture depends on yourself and how badly you want it. Regular exercise, going to the gym, or working with a personal trainer can speed up the process. If you find it hard to correct your body posture on your own, it may be a wise decision to visit the chiropractor to see if there are easier ways.

Walking or sitting a certain way for years may have pulled muscles into the wrong positions. Sometimes our muscles have lost its strength or shape because of bad posture and not enough exercising. The vertebrae could also have moved slightly, that will need a chiropractor's help to correct. Through persevering every day, you will be able to change your posture and eventually reap all the benefits of it. A beautiful and upright body posture is key to looking and feeling younger for longer in life. It not only gives you a beautiful appearance, but also let you appear younger and more energetic.

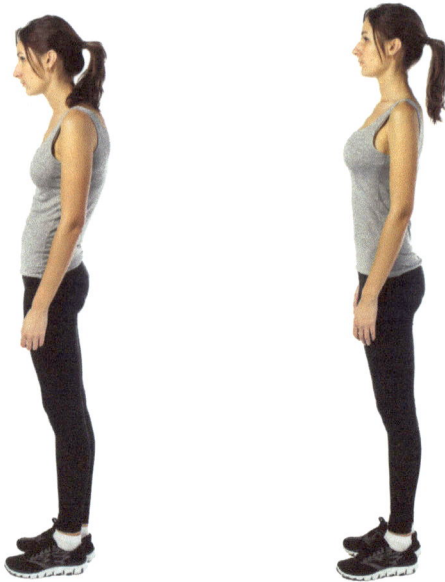

Bad posture verses good posture

Technology has advanced so quickly over the past thirty years that our lives have become fast-paced, with knowledge at our fingertips. Unfortunately with smart phones and tablets in the picture, young and old are spending hours a day on them, therefore we are running the risk of a huge health epidemic in the years to come, if we are complacent about this. Sitting or lying down with our head tilted and looking at the phone or tablet's screens will affect our posture in the decades to come. Spending hours on phones and tablets takes most children and adults away from spending valuable time in the sun and nature, causing Vitamin D deficiency. But most catastrophically, it takes people away from exercising that keeps muscles strong, and the spine and bones in the correct alignment. Even eyes will be affected and more people will require reading glasses sooner in life.

These negative results are discussed regularly on television programs and in magazines, but most people decide to ignore them. There is a feeling of, if it is not broken, why fix it. I would like to encourage every reader to start making an informed decision to cut down on the time spent on the internet and social media. Work movement, exercise and nature into your weeks. Ensure you have that balance in your life to include everything mentioned in this book for a healthy body and mentally strong mind. Those with a healthy body and mind are the ones who will look and feel younger for longer. A healthy body and mind will also keep a person positive, which again produces a healthier and happier life.

HAIR CARE

As explained in the beginning of this book, your hair is part of your face, and also helps to create your identity. You can have the most beautiful facial features, be well-dressed, and wear make-up; but if your hair is oily and not well cared for, it will be a drawback in your overall appearance. Oily hair can even make you look ill or tired. Grooming and the styling of our hair play a huge role in our general sense of attractiveness. If a woman's hair is well-groomed, she's more confident and does not need to wear a lot of make-up. Even men will have that extra boost of confidence if they know their hair looks good.

I also want to draw your attention again to the fact that you have to be content with what you are born with, and make the best of what you have. The majority of women are not happy with their hair and want to change it continuously. I found that it is because of this attitude that they do more harm than good to their hair. Let me explain what I mean. Some women born with black or brown hair want blonde hair, and they will bleach their hair, making it look dull, dry and brittle. Others with blonde hair want black hair. Although this is not that bad as chemical treatment like bleaching, it still lifts up the cuticles of the hair to push in the black colour, making the hair more porous. Women with thin hair want thick hair, and use regular teasing to give it body. Some also attach hair extensions to their hair to build the volume of their hair, where the glues and clips again break their natural hair. And women with thick hair want less hair. People always desire to look like others who they admire, and forget that each of us are unique and has our own characteristics. We waste our money and time by spending hours a day to change who we are. Do you understand what I am saying?

I have naturally curly hair, and as I get older it becomes frizzier. When I was younger I spent hours straightening it, till I realised that the amount of time I spent on my hair, and the damage I caused to my hair were not worth it. I got to the point where I realised I have to change my attitude by accepting who God has made me to be. Only at that moment I started to be happier with my hair. The best outcome with this change of mindset was that I had more time for myself to grow mentally, spiritually and in knowledge. Now let me get more into the physics of hair.

ORIGIN OF HUMAN HAIR

- By week 22, a developing foetus has all of its hair follicles formed. This is the largest number of hair follicles a human will ever have, since we do not generate new hair follicles anytime during the course of our lifetime.

- There are between 1-5 million follicles on a human body, with 90,000 to 150,000 of those follicles residing on the scalp. Blondes have an average of 150,000 hairs on their head, black or brown hair averages 100,000 to 110,000 hairs, and red heads have an average of 90,000 hairs.

- Another difference in hair is the diameter of the hair and of course the shape of the follicles in the head. A curvy shaped follicle will produce curly hair.

- Most people will notice that the density of the hair on their scalp is reduced as they grow from childhood to adulthood. The reason is that our scalp expands as we grow.

Redheads have a lower amount of hair on their scalp because red hair has generally a greater hair diameter See the sketch below showing the three diameters of hair.

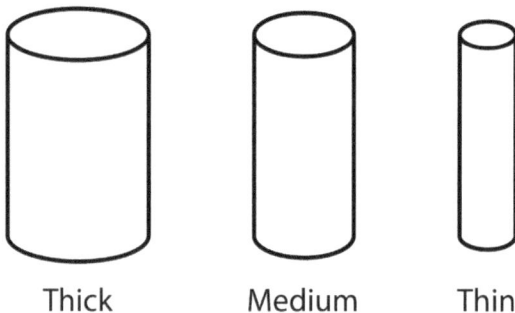

Thick   Medium   Thin

The shape of your hair is determined by the shape of the hair follicle in the scalp. See the sketch below.

SHAPE OF THE HAIR

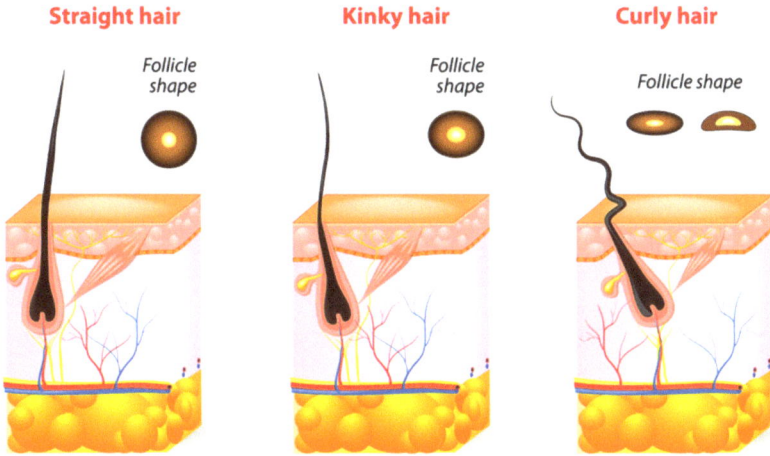

Straight hair

Follicle shape

Kinky hair

Follicle shape

Curly hair

Follicle shape

THE HAIR GROWTH CYCLE

Here is the *Hair Growth Cycle* explained so you can understand why you have at certain times less hair on your head, and other times more hair. It will also explain why you have lost your hair, and why you have trouble growing your hair. Hair grows in three stages. The first stage is called the anagen stage or growth phase, the second stage is the catagen stage or transition phase, and the third stage is the telogen stage or resting phase.

Anagen Stage –The hair growth phase

- Hair grows around 1.25 cm per month.

- The Growth or Anagen stage lasts an average of 3-5 years, full-length hair averages 45 – 76cm.

- The Anagen stage is generally longer in Asians, and can last as long as 7 years with hair being able to grow to 1 metre. It is for this reason why Asian hair is popular to use in the making of wigs.

Catagen Stage – Transition phase

- At the end of the Anagen stage, your hair enters the Catagen stage.

- The hair follicle detaches from the nourishing blood supply and hair growth stops.

- Now the hair follicle itself shrinks rapidly, pushing the hair upwards, and the strand of hair can be easily shed through normal activity.

- This transition phase can last approximately 1-2 weeks.

Telogen Stage – Resting phase

- This is the resting phase when hair is released and falls out.

- The follicle then remains inactive for three months and the whole process is repeated.

- Each hair follicle is independent and goes through the growth cycle at different times. That is why your hair is thicker at some stages.

HAIR GROWTH CYCLE

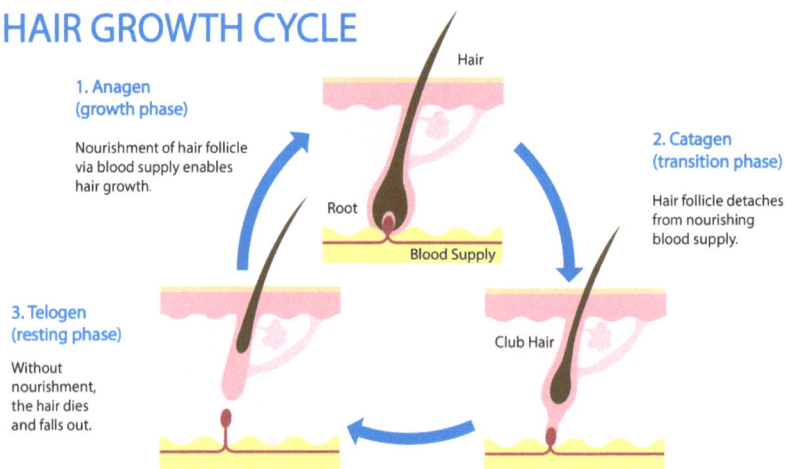

Hair

1. Anagen (growth phase)

Nourishment of hair follicle via blood supply enables hair growth.

Root

Blood Supply

2. Catagen (transition phase)

Hair follicle detaches from nourishing blood supply.

Club Hair

3. Telogen (resting phase)

Without nourishment, the hair dies and falls out.

You shed a certain number of hairs a day, between 50-100 hairs on a healthy head. Hair loss, hair thinning and problems with hair growth, occur when your growth cycle is disrupted. This can be triggered by conditions such as metabolic imbalances, illness or improper nutrition.

REASONS FOR HAIR LOSS

- Shedding hair is different from hair loss. Shedding hair is a natural process as described in the hair growth cycle; where the hair does grow back during the cycle.

- Hair loss is when hair falls out due to a problem or sickness.

- Alopecia is the term for baldness. It can be a partial or complete absence of hair from some areas of the body or head where it normally grows.

- Six weeks after a restrictive dieting or a fever you can experience Telogen Effluvium (diffuse hair falls). In most cases this occurs when the Anagen or growth phase is cut short, and many hairs enter the Telogen or resting phase all at the same time.

- If your hair growth cycle is constantly challenged, or not supported, you may find that your hair won't grow as long as it used to.

CONDITION OF HAIR

FIGURE 1   FIGURE 2   FIGURE 3

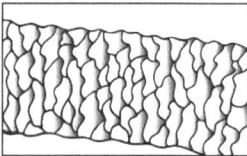 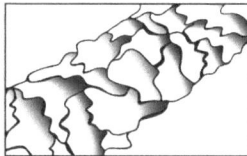 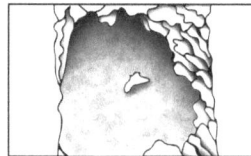

FIGURE 1 - Hair is healthy and smooth, the scales are closed.
FIGURE 2 - Hair is porous and scales are raised.
FIGURE 3 - Damaged hair with missing scales. Damaged hair cannot be repaired. A trim is the only way to revive damaged hair.

Hair gets damaged by hair chemicals, too-warm air from the hairdryer, hot styling tools, teasing of hair, cutting the hair with blunt scissors, tying the hair too tightly with elastics, pool chemicals, the wrong shampoo and conditioner, the wrong way of blow drying the hair, washing the hair in too hot water, swimming regularly in the sea's salty water. All these processes have an influence on the condition of our hair. Some people may have more of the mentioned causes combined that can really damage the hair beyond repair. In the summer months we enjoy the sun, regular dips in the pool or salty sea water. But before going for a swim, you can moisten your hair completely, and thoroughly applying a leave-in conditioner. Your hair will then absorb the conditioner instead of the chlorine or salt water.

Another issue that most people do not even know about is that hair can get easily damaged while we sleep on our pillow every night for six to eight hours. Hair damage is caused while we sleep due to the hair being roughed up and tangled. A silk pillow will help give a more slippery surface for the hair to avoid excess friction. Never go to sleep with hair clips, elastics, or bobby pins in your hair.

I do not recommend that you use hot styling tools on your hair every day, because your hair will not withstand this harsh treatment. Keep that for special occasions. When you are using hot styling tools on your hair like a straightener, hot curlers, or curling tongs, please buy a heat protecting leave-in hair product that will shield the hair a bit from the heat, providing some level of protection. Also make sure the hot styling hair tools are not too hot because you can damage the hair so badly with just one treatment. The next important thing to remember is to always work with the hair cuticles and not against them. For example, do not blow dry the hair upwards so that the air lifts the cuticles of the hair. Blow dry at ninety degrees or down onto the hair, so that the cuticles stay closed, protecting the hair from dehydration. Never slide a hot straightener in an upward motion that will lift the hair cuticles and most likely break it off instantly.

Bleaching all your hair is a definite 'no' in my view, as you'll never get your hair healthy after that, except for the new hair that grows out. Bleaching to give your hair highlights and lowlights are professional services that need to be done by a professional who knows what they are doing. I recommend that you go to a hairdresser if you want to add highlights or lowlights, who can do it professionally for you. This will be less damaging if done correctly.

One can pick a professional hair colour treatment from a home colour treatment straight away. It takes only one wrong chemical treatment to your hair to make it look lifeless or damaged. If you are a person who likes to experiment with different hairdos, experiment with different modern haircuts, hair gels, and different blow drying techniques, rather than bleaching your hair, as this may take years to correct or grow out to look healthy again. Doing your own bleaching and hair colour at home and not knowing how to do it professionally can make your hair look dull and even cheap. Alternatively you can buy a couple of natural hair wigs to give that different look every time, and your own hair will stay healthy.

Each person needs to be responsible for looking after their hair and giving it daily or at least weekly treatments, to maintain it and keep it healthy. You can use organic coconut oil to massage your scalp twice a week for two-five minutes that will increase hair growth, making it stronger and dandruff free. Leave the coconut oil in for a few hours or even overnight to feed the hair. But sleep on a towel then not to rub off the oil on your pillowcase and pillow. To remove most of the oil, wash your scalp with lukewarm to warm water and shampoo. Never use too warm or hot water to remove the oil because it can undo the good treatment you just gave your hair. Do not worry about removing all the oil as it will give your hair some shine for the next day or so, and will eventually wash out. A hot shower is not good for you hair or skin, but if you do like more of a hot shower, wash your hair separately in a washbasin or with a mixer over the bath or shower. This will prevent you from removing all the natural oil the scalp is producing to feed and protect the hair. Those with naturally oily hair must not feed the hair with more oil though. If the ends are dry, just feed the ends.

Be mindful not to walk around for days without washing your scalp, because a build-up of natural oil excretion from the hair follicles will give your hair an oily look, and a bad odour. When washing your hair, you really have to wash the scalp and the rest of the hair will automatically be cleansed. The mistake that a lot of women and men make who have long hair is, to start washing the long strands of hair rather than their scalp. This is why their hair will look oily at day two or three. Notice when you go to the hairdresser which part of the hair they'll mostly wash. They primarily wash the scalp and the rest of the hair will be cleansed in the process.

All dryness of hair is a result of wind, sun (direct sunlight), heat (curling tongs, straighteners, hot water, blow dryers), harsh water (tap, pool or sea water), chemical processes (highlighting, low lights, colouring, perming and bleaching). One myth that I want to make you aware of as well is the idea that hair growth cannot be stimulated or increased by shaving, cutting, clipping or singeing.

Nourishment of Hair

Hair is reproduced and grows within the skin. The hair that emerges from the skin no longer grows. Therefore the health of the hair depends upon the nourishment it receives before it grows from the follicle, i.e. the hair root is nourished by the bloodstream. That is why your diet is very important in having healthy hair.

How do you test if your hair is healthy?
Healthy hair is hydrated and has a beautiful shine to it. The cuticles of the hair are closed, giving it a smooth look and feel. When you take a strand of hair and pull it from either side, it should not break immediately. If it does break, that's a sign of unhealthy hair. Hair that is healthy is elastic and will stretch a bit like an elastic band, but will return to its original form.

Combing or brushing your hair every day has a lot of health benefits for your hair. It stimulates the scalp that helps to increase blood flow. The increased circulation brings with it more oxygen and nutrients to the hair, which nourishes the hair roots and promotes hair growth. Combing or brushing also activates the sebaceous glands to the scalp's natural oil.

THE DIFFERENT HAIR TYPES

As we all have different skin types, there are also four different hair types that hair can fall into. The four different hair types are as follows:

Normal hair

- Looks shiny and lustrous.
- It feels smooth and supple.
- When stretched, it returns to its original form.

Oily hair

- Appears oily to the eye.
- It feels oily and greasy.
- When stretched, it returns to its original form.

Dry hair

- Slightly dry – May be shiny and naturally looking. By feel it will be soft and perhaps little dry.
- Moderately dry – Hair will look dull, feel dry & may lack elasticity.
- Very dry – Hair looks dull, will be rough & 'straw like', and lacks elasticity.

Damaged hair

- Hair looks spongy and tangled when hair is wet.
- Coloured hair fades quickly or it absorbs too much colour in hair colouring processes.

- Hair has a rough structure.

- Hair is very dry and largely porous.

- It has no elasticity and is easy to break.

- Hair is a lot of times so damaged and cannot be repaired with any topical hair products. In this case the best will be to cut it and grow out healthier hair.

Once hair has emerged from the scalp, it can be nourished through a topical way:

- Shampoo and conditioners for the specific hair type or condition.

- Hair masks that treat for the specific hair condition.

- Massage the scalp with coconut oil for 2-5 minutes, twice a week.

- Stop the harming treatments for a while caused by electrical curlers and straighteners.

Tips to keep your hair healthy and shiny:

1. Do not wash your hair under a hot shower. Wash your hair in a washbasin or shower head with cold to lukewarm water. Cold water is the best, but depending on the season of the year. Cold water during winter time is not pleasant.

2. Deep condition your hair once a week with a hair mask, repair conditioner, or coconut oil. The secret is to leave it in for 5-15 minutes before rinsing it off.

3. Apply a heat protecting lotion before drying your hair that will protect your hair from heat coming from a hairdryer, straighteners or curling tongs.

4. After you have blow-dried your hair, use the cool air button on the hairdryer to cool down the hair. This will help close the hair cuticles, making it stronger and shinier.

5. Take breaks in blow drying your hair during the week and let it dry on its own. You can even stand outside in the sun for 15 minutes to let it dry while combing it with a wide-tooth comb a few times. If the wind is too wild, it is best not to stand outside to dry, because your hair will get tangled and cause breakages while you try to de-tangle it. Standing for 15 minutes in normal strength sunrays will also help you get your Vitamin D dose for the day as well. Do not attempt this in the cold winter month resulting in catching a cold or worse.

6. Your hair is the most vulnerable when it is wet, therefore use a wide-tooth comb to comb the conditioner through. Refrain from brushing your hair with a normal hairbrush when it is wet, because it will cause hair breakage easily.

7. Eat a healthy diet every day to give your hair the best nutrients to grow strong and healthy from the inside.

8. Long hair must get a trim at least every 3-6 months to get rid of the split ends so that the hair looks healthier. A trim can only be 5mm (0.5cm) to cut off the dry and split ends if you are in the process of growing your hair.

9. Stay away from harsh treatments like perms, bleaching, and cutting with blunt scissors. Use hair scissors only and not paper scissors.

MY QUICK REFERENCE GUIDE

1. What are the extrinsic factors or external factors that I can control in my life to help me looking younger for longer in life? (Refer to page 16)

_____

_____

_____

_____

2. How can I improve in my every day skin practices to cleanse my face and neck the correct way? (Refer to pages 21-23)

_____

_____

_____

_____

3. My skin type is: (Refer to page 24) _____

4. The best types of face and neck cleansers to use for my skin type and lifestyle are:

(Refer to page 26-27)

_____   _____

_____   _____

_____   _____

5. Things that I must focus on to look after my face and neck better:

(Refer to page 33)

Do's: _____

_____

_____

Don'ts: _____

_____

_____

6. My face and neck cleansing steps in short:

(Refer to pages 34-38 for women and pages 39-44 for men)

STEP 1: _____

STEP 2: _____

STEP 3: _____

STEP 4: _____

STEP 5: _____

STEP 6: _____

STEP 7: _____

7. My child under 10 years' face and neck cleansing steps in short:

(Refer to pages 44–47)

STEP 1: _____

STEP 2: _____

STEP 3: _____

STEP 4: _____

8. The ideal skin care routine for women and men in a Weekly table:

Day	Steps for Morning Procedure	Steps for Night Procedure
Sunday	1. Cleansing 2. Skin toner 3. Eye cream 4. Moisturiser with a SPF*	1. Cleansing 2. **Gentle exfoliating** 3. **Mask** 4. Skin toner 5. Eye cream 6. Moisturiser / night cream
Monday	1. Cleansing 2. Skin toner 3. Eye cream 4. Moisturiser with a SPF*	1. Cleansing 2. Skin toner 3. Eye cream 4. Moisturiser / night cream
Tuesday	1. Cleansing 2. Skin toner 3. Eye cream 4. Moisturiser with a SPF*	1. Cleansing 2. Skin toner 3. Eye cream 4. Moisturiser / night cream
Wednesday	1. Cleansing 2. Skin toner 3. Eye cream 4. Moisturiser with a SPF*	1. Cleansing 2. **Gentle exfoliating** 3. **Mask** 4. Skin Toner 5. Eye cream 6. Moisturiser / night cream
Thursday	1. Cleansing 2. Skin toner 3. Eye cream 4. Moisturiser with a SPF*	1. Cleansing 2. Skin toner 3. Eye cream 4. Moisturiser / night cream
Friday	1. Cleansing 2. Skin toner 3. Eye cream 4. Moisturiser with a SPF*	1. Cleansing 2. Skin toner 3. Eye cream 4. Moisturiser / night cream
Saturday	1. Cleansing 2. Skin toner 3. Eye cream 4. Moisturiser with a SPF*	1. Cleansing 2. Skin toner 3. Eye cream 4. Moisturiser / night cream

9. How long can I stay in the sun for, before I'll burn my skin: (refer to page 53)

It takes me $\boxed{10}$ $\boxed{15}$ $\boxed{20}$ $\boxed{25}$ minutes for my skin to show redness.

Use this equation to work it out

MINUTES YOU BURN WITHOUT SUNSCREEN X SPF NUMBER
= MAXIMUM SUN EXPOSURE TIME

SPF 15 _____

SPF 30 _____

SPF 50 _____

10. What do the following symbols on the packaging of skin product and cosmetics mean? (Refer to page 59)

6 M _____

12 M _____

24 M _____

11. Simple home remedies for the face and neck are on pages 63-72

    Which remedies will work best for my skin type?

    _____ it is on page _____

    _____ it is on page _____

    _____ it is on page _____

12. Foods that I eat that may cause inflammation in my body? (Refer to pages 96-99)

13. What do I want to change in my every day diet? (Refer to pages 96-108)

To gain your self-confidence through how you style,
the book *Style Yourself with Confidence*
by Ellen Joubert is a must read.

It is available in hard cover, soft cover, and eBook.

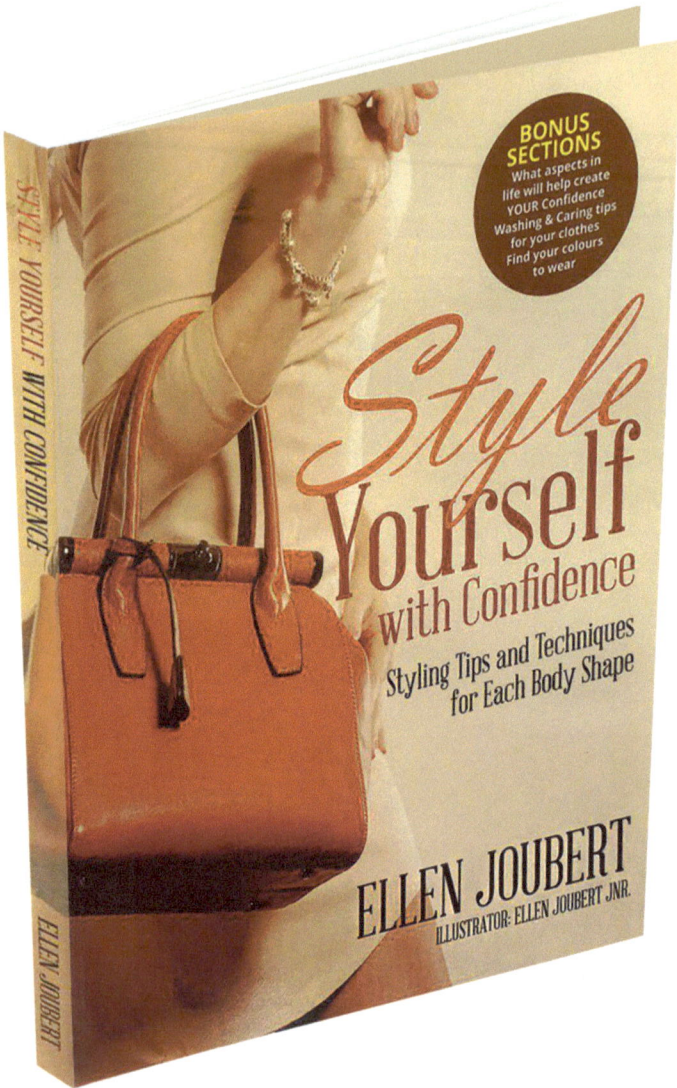

With **255 beautiful illustrations and colour images**,
this book is a practical application for all women, teaching
them how to style their specific features the best.

STYLE YOURSELF
WITH CONFIDENCE
Styling Tips and Techniques for Each Body Shape

The purpose of this book is to make it easy for every woman to understand the art of being well-dressed and to have a practical application on how to emphasise her good features and hide or minimise the less attractive ones. Gaining knowledge on the correct way to dress will make so much more sense when buying clothes and styling yourself every day. Well-dressed women stand out from the crowd and attract good attention. They have loads of confidence and the term 'confident in her own skin' comes to mind.

Good style does not come naturally to most of us. We are not born with good style genes. There are a lot of factors involved in our dress style, and one of them is education.

Once you have the understanding of how clothing styles and colour work, you'll be enlightened for the rest of your life. You'll even be a role model for your children and grandchildren.

The good news is you do not have to buy your clothes only at high-end boutiques to make an impression. Everyday styles will work well if you know the tricks of how to bring out the best of your own body shape and features. Since a woman can have two to three different body shapes during her lifetime, this book will be a lifetime investment. We are never too young or too old to learn about style secrets and how to dress stylishly. The information in this book is suitable for women of all ages.

Mothers, even your teenage daughters will benefit from reading this book. The sooner they gain confidence in style, the sooner they'll be set on the road of being stylish and successful.

To help every woman make an overall transformation in her appearance and self-confidence, this book includes bonus sections such as: 'Find your colours to wear', 'How to choose your shoes', 'Choose the best frame for your face shape', all aspects that will help increase your self-confidence in life.

BIBLIOGRAPHY

121 Dietician, 'Salt Awareness Week: Sea Salt & Rock Salt -Healthier Options?', www.121dietitian.com, Web, 22 February 2018.

ABC Health & Wellbeing, 'How much sun do you need?', www.abc.net.au, Web, 1 March 2018.

Adelaja, Ayo, 'Understanding Why Being Positive Is Important', www.theodysseyonline.com, Web,16 February 2018.

American Board of Cosmetic Surgery, 'Cosmetic Surgery vs. Plastic Surgery', www.americanboardcosmeticsurgery.org, Web, 9 March 2018.

Andreeva, Nadya, '10 Common Food Combinations That Wreak Havoc on Your Health', www.mindbodygreen.com, Web, 26 February 2018.

Ask women net. 'The Factors of Skin Aging'. www.askwomennet.com,Web, 2 February 2018.

Barret-Hill, Florence, 'Skin differences beyond colour alone', www.beautymagonline .com1, Web, 2 March 2018.

Benvenuti, Nicki Zevola, '5 Important Reasons You Must Cleanse Your Face Morning and Night', www.futurederm.com, Web,12 February 2018.

Boztas, Senay, Facial Filler Injections, www.independent.co.uk , Web, 9 March 2018.

Brind'Amour, Katherine, Healthline, 'Common Skin Disorders', www.healthline.com, Web,14 February 2018.

Carmody, Ryan, 'The Truth About Food Combining and Smoothies', www.healthysmoothiehq.com, Web, 26 February 2018.

Cleveland Clinic, 'How Ultrasound Skin Tightening Can Firm, Lift Your Face', www.health.clevelandclinic.org, Web, 9 March 2018.

Coco ruby Skin and Anti-Ageing, 'Facial Fillers: The Ugly Truth about Permanent Facial Fillers', www.cocorubyskin.com.au, Web, 9 March 2018.

Cooper, Allison, Reader's Digest, 'This Is What Your Doctor REALLY Thinks of Those Trending Facial Exercises', www.rd.com, Web,14 March 2018.

Cosmetic Calculator, 'Cosmetic shelf life F.A.Q.', [website], www.checkcosmetic.net, Web, 12 February 2018.

Davis, Jeanie, 'Salt: Don't Ban It Entirely', www.webmd.com, Web,22 February 2018.

Dr. Colbert's Keto Zone Diet, eBook, pages: 33-36,

Dr. Gloria Klein, 'Face Up with Anneline Kriel', book accessed in 1990.

Dr. Kaslow, 'Food Combining', www.drkaslow.com, Web, 28 February.

Drugs.com, 'What is Botox?', www.drugs.com, Web, 9 March 2018.

Encyclopaedia Britannica, 'Human Skin Anatomy', www.britannica.com, Web, 10 February 2018.

Harvard men's health watch. 'Vitamin D and your health: Breaking old rules, raising new hopes' www.health.harvard.edu/newsletter. Web. 2 February 2018.

Haslett, Sophie, 'Revealed: The simple mistake you're making every day when washing your face that is DESTROYING your skin', Web, www.dailymail.co.uk, Web,10 February 2018.

Heathman, Christine, 'The Physiology of Skin of Color', www.dermascope.com, Web, 12 March 2018.

Heritage Integrative Healthcare, *The Importance of Chewing Your Food',* www.heritageihc.com, Web,15 February 2018.

Hofweber, Anne, 'Why Is Drinking Cold Water Bad For You?', www.curejoy.com, Web, 20 February 2018.

Hyman, Mark, 'Three Hidden Ways Wheat Makes You Fat', www.drhyman.com, Web, 1 August 2018.

Jackson, C. Color Me Beautiful, Discover Your Natural Beauty through Colours That Make You Look Great and Feel Fabulous (Washington D.C. Acropolis Books Ltd, 1980), p. 78.

Jackson, C. Color Me Beautiful, Discover Your Natural Beauty through Colours That Make You Look Great and Feel Fabulous (Washington D.C. Acropolis Books Ltd, 1980), 'Posture', page 78, accessed 3 May 2018.

Kukreja, Kushneet, '20 Effective Home Remedies For Glowing Skin That Really Work', www.stylecraze.com, Web, 9 March 2018.

Labiberte, Marissa, Reader's Digest, '13 Surprising Home Remedies for Acne', www.rd.com, Web,12 March 2018.

Leech, Joe, '11 Proven Health Benefits of Ginger', www.healthline.com, Web, 4 March 2018.

Leech, Joe, '10 Evidence-Based Health Benefits of Cinnamon', www.healthline.com, Web, 4 March 2018.

Lose baby weight, 'What Happens If You Eat Too Much Wheat', www.losebabyweight.com.au, Web, 1 August 2018.

Miss Craig', 'Face Saving Exercises', book accessed in 1990.

Naish, John, 'How cosmetic fillers can destroy your looks', www.dailymail.co.uk, Web, 9 March 2018.

Nall, Rachel, 'Muscle Tension From Lack of Exercise', www.livestrong.com, Web, 16 February 2018.

Nordqvist, Christian, 'Salt: Do we really need it, and how much should we eat?', www.medicalnewstoday.com, Web, 22 February 2018.

Pesticide Action Network UK, ' 'Promoting safe and sustainable alternatives to hazardous pesticides', www.pan-uk.org/, Web, 2 June 2018.

Raw Food explained, 'Harmful Drinking Practices', www.rawfoodexplained.com, Web, 21 February 2018.

Reference. 'Why is skin considered an organ?', IAC Publishing, www.reference. com. Web. 2 February 2018.

RICHFEEL Hair Doctors to the Nation, 'Does Your Hair Really Undergo Changes On Regular Basis?', www.richfeel.com, Web, 7 May, 2018.

Skin Cancer Foundation, 'UVA & UVB', www.skincancer.org, Web, 28 February 2018.

Skinbotanica, 'Balancing Act! pH Balance of Skin', www.skincarerx.com, Web, 10 February 2018.

Steen, Juliette, 'We Found Out What 'Food Combining' Is (And If It Actually Works)', www.huffingtonpost.com.au, Web, 20 February 2018.

Tarrantino, Olivia, '14 Inflammatory Foods Making You Fat', www.eatthis. com, Web, 3 June 2018.

The Conversation, 'A history of sugar – the food nobody needs, but everyone craves', www.theconversation.com, Web, 15 February 2018.

The science of eating, '10 Foods You Should Not Eat Together', www.thescien-ceofeating.com, Web, 26 February 2018.

Vakil, Enzio, 5 food combinations that could make you sick', www.digitaljour-nal.com, Web, 28 February 2018.

Warner, Jennifer, 'Laser Resurfacing: Lasting Wrinkle Fix?', www.webmd .com, Web, March 2018.

WebMD, 'Your Digestive System', *[website]*, www.webmd.com, Web, 14 February 2018.

Whiterskin, 'Black skin, white skin, Asian skin – what's the difference?',www. whiterskin.info, Web, 12 March 2018.

Wikipedia The Free Encyclopedia, 'Facial rejuvenation', <https://en. wikipedia.org, Web, 9 March 2018.

Wikipedia The Free Encyclopedia, 'Human skin color', https://en. wikipedia.org, Web, 12 March 2018.

Wikipedia The Free Encyclopedia, 'Photorejuvenation', https://en. wikipedia.org , Web, 9 March 2018.

Wikipedia The Free Encyclopedia, 'Radio frequency skin tightening', https:// en.wikipedia.org, Web, 9 March 2018.

Wikipedia. 'Human skin' en.wikipedia.org. Web. 2 February 2018.

Zimmerman, Kim, 'Lymphatic System: Facts, Functions & Diseases', www. livescience.com, Web, 8 June 2018.

Shutterstock Images Used in this Book:

And-One, *'Mother teaching her young son how to wash his face in the bathroom - Royalty-free stock photo ID: 1052861885'*, Web, 30 June 2018.

Anna Ok, *'Rose attar cleaning tonic water fresh flower white cotton pads and towel, empty space, soft focus, bathroom daily care - Royalty-free stock photo ID: 316143185'*, Web, 30 June 2018.

Antonova Ganna, *'Sliced banana in bowl on white wooden background. Selective focus - Royalty-free stock photo ID: 186391109'*, Web, 30 June 2018.

DenisProduction.com, *'Girl wearing collagen mask. Radio frequency skin tightening, face - Royalty-free stock photo ID: 704647351'*, Web, 30 June 2018.

Designua, *'Healthy skin and Blackheads - Royalty-free stock vector ID: 407925238'*, Web, 8 May 2018.

Designua, *'Structure of the Human skin. Anatomy diagram. different cell types populating the skin –Royalty-free stock illustration ID: 251498023'*, Web, 29 September 2017.

Designua, *'types of hair. Cross section of different hair texture. Follicle shape determines hair texture. Straight, wavy, curly, kinky and spiral hair - Royalty-free stock vector ID: 161871173'*, Web, 30 June 2018.

Geo-grafika, *'Close-up of baking soda in a glass jar. Bicarbonate of soda - Royalty-free stock photo ID: 179857913'*, Web, 30 June 2018.

Iryna Denysova, *'Top view of white bowl of olive oil,and towel decorated with green olive fruit isolated on white background. Hands Spa. Manicure concept - Royalty-free stock photo ID: 478213126'*, Web, 30 June 2018.

KMNPhoto, *'healthy green tea cup with tea leaves - Royalty-free stock photo ID: 146183111'*, Web, 30 June 2018.

Kraska, *'Sun Cream Containers. Vector illustration - Royalty-free stock vector ID: 72011293'*, Web, 30 June 2018.

La Gorda, *'Human digestive system vector illustration - Royalty-free stock vector ID: 153338039'*, Web, 30 June 2018.

Leonid and Anna Dedukh, *'portrait of attractive caucasian smiling woman isolated on white studio shot washing her face - Royalty-free stock photo ID: 94252843'*, Digital Image, Web, 30 June 2018.

And-One, *'Man washing his face in the bathroom sink - Royalty-free stock photo ID: 370518860'*, Web, 30 June 2018.

MK photograp55, *'aloe vera gel on wooden spoon with aloe vera on wooden table - Royalty-free stock photo ID: 301572848'*, Web, 30 June 2018.

Nata-Lia, *'coconut and oil - Royalty-free stock photo ID: 169315001'*, Web, 30 June 2018.

Nataly Studio, *'Bottle of almond oil and almonds in a wooden bowl isolated on white background - Royalty-free stock photo ID: 678364822'*, Web, 30 June 2018.

Nattha99, *'makeup sponge isolated on white background -Royalty-free stock photo ID: 1006872790'*, Web, 30 June 2018.

Oksana Shevchenko, *'Pieces of honeycomb with spoon and glass jar with honey are on a wooden board. Outdoor background - Royalty-free stock photo ID: 532752952'*, Web, 30 June 2018.

Robert Przybysz, *'Cavitation peeling, handsome man with a beautician for the treatment of facial skin - Royalty-free stock photo ID: 231818134'*, Web, 30 June 2018.

Tefi, *'Muscles of the face and the name of each muscle, detailed bright anatomy isolated on a white background - Royalty-free stock vector ID: 792337048'*, Web, 30 June 2018.

TR Growth, *'The pH scale Universal Indicator pH Color Chart diagram acidic alkaline values common substances vector illustration flat icon design Colorful'*, Royalty-free stock vector ID: 674361793, Web, 8 May 2018.

Undrey, *'Woman with impaired posture position defect scoliosis and ideal bearing - Royalty-free stock photo ID: 265889168'*, Web, 2 June 2017.

Valentina Proskurina, *'Fresh raw mint leaves isolated on white background - Royalty-free stock photo ID: 154608077'*, Web, 30 June 2018.

Wavebreakmedia, *'Close-up of sugar written on sugar powder on table - Royalty-free stock photo ID: 516079558'*, Web, 30 June 2018.

Yomogi1, *'infographic skin illustration. UVA and UVB penetration into the human skin. sunscreen protect the skin from radiation - Royalty-free stock vector ID: 597626417'*, Web, 30 June 2018.

Yuriy Maksymiv, *'Cosmetology. Procedure of Microdermabrasion. Mechanical Exfoliation, diamond polishing. Model and doctor. Cosmetological clinic. Healthcare, clinic, cosmetology. High Resolution - Royalty-free stock photo ID: 599185625'*, Web, 30 June 2018.

www.ingramcontent.com/pod-product-compliance
Lightning Source LLC
Chambersburg PA
CBHW040932030426
42336CB00001B/1